D0426672

THE HUMAN GENOME PROJECT

Cracking the Genetic Code of Life

THE HUMAN GENOME PROJECT

Cracking the Genetic Code of Life

Thomas F. Lee

Plenum Press • New York and London

Library of Congress Cataloging-in-Publication Data

Lee, Thomas F., Ph. D.
    The Human Genome Project : cracking the genetic code of life /
  Thomas F. Lee.
        p.   cm.
    Includes bibliographical references and index.
    ISBN 0-306-43965-4
    1. Human Genome Project.   I. Title.
    [DNLM: 1. Human Genome Project.   2. Chromosome Mapping.
  3. Genome, Human.   QH 447 L481h]
  QH447.L44   1991
  573.2'12--dc20
  DNLM/DLC
  for Library of Congress   91-21358
                                                                 CIP

First Printing — August 1991
Second Printing — November 1992

ISBN 0-306-43965-4

© 1991 Thomas F. Lee
Plenum Press is a division of Plenum Publishing Corporation
233 Spring Street, New York, N.Y. 10013

Printed in the United States of America

ACKNOWLEDGMENTS

I would like to thank my many colleagues who offered their advice and encouragement during the writing of this book. I am particularly grateful to Karen Metz, Dennis Berthiaume, and Jeanne Welch of the Geisel Library staff for their gracious assistance in the research phase. Thanks also to Sandra Reichenbach for her meticulous secretarial help and to Dr. James McGhee for his wise advice on questions of ethics. Rich DeScenzo was, as usual, most generous with his knowledge on matters of molecular biology. My daughter Anne typed beyond the call of duty and Jill Osburn worked diligently on the illustrations as did Jeff Thibodeau of Graphics House. Jeff's timely and expert cooperation is gratefully acknowledged. My work could not have been completed without the loving generosity of my wife Eileen and my children Anne, Brian, Emily, Julie, Bridget, and Rebecca. And finally, a special nod to Professor John Feick, without whose input the finished product would have been considerably different.

CONTENTS

1

THE JOURNEY BEGINS

A scientific research effort is currently under way which is unlike anything ever before attempted. International in its scope, it is enormously expensive and, if successful, could lead to our ultimate control of human disease, aging, and death. It is nothing short of a revolution against the way science has traditionally progressed. The plans have ignited fervent enthusiasm among many in the scientific community; others have attacked it as wildly optimistic. It has come to be known as the Human Genome Project (HGP), and its findings may radically change and enrich our lives, while opening up a bewildering array of serious ethical dilemmas.

The goal of this project is nothing less than determining the precise location and molecular details of all of the genes and interconnecting segments which make up the human chromosomes. Since genes are the tiny but complex chemical segments that control the activities of the cells and hence those of the entire organism, such knowledge would be an extraordinarily powerful tool to explore what are now unfathomable mysteries of human development and disease.

In the following pages we will explore the methods and significance of this awesome undertaking and tell the tale of the personalities, institutions, and controversies involved. The extraordinary developments beginning as recently as 1970 that have led to the possibility of even conceiving of such a project will be explained as well. We hope to bridge the gap between the arcane world of the laboratory scientist and the experience of those of our readers not necessarily formally trained in the biological sciences, whose lives are even now being changed by these genetic studies.

In order to relate the relatively brief but convoluted genesis of the HGP, we must first adequately define the term *genome*. It means simply the total of an individual's genetic material, that part of her or his cells that controls her or his heredity. We also need to explain why an intimate understanding of the human genome under the rubric of the HGP has become so central in the pantheon of modern biology.

The life sciences are no longer confined to the study of the more obvious characteristics of plants and animals such as their anatomy or their various living functions like feeding, mobility, and sexual reproduction. As the technology supporting scientific investigation has developed and landmark discoveries have been made, the scale of the details of living organisms that have been studied and analyzed has been enormously extended. It ranges all the way from the large and small structures visible to the naked eye, to those available through the light microscope, and finally to the view afforded by the ultimate weapon, the electron microscope, with which one can literally see molecules.

The study of human *heredity*, that set of events that determines how characteristics are passed from generation to generation and around which the HGP is centered, has likewise proceeded from studies of the inheritance pattern within the familiar family tree to the minute details of the hereditary units nestled within the nuclei of our cells—the chromosomes.

Within these coiled strands lies the key to all that an organism is and does. An understanding of how our chromosomes are designed and why they are so vitally important is essential to appreciating the irresistible lure of uncovering their most minute details.

Looking into a light microscope at a preserved, stained, squashed human cell (white blood cells are routinely used for this) one can see 46 dark threadlike objects. These are the chromosomes, long, tightly coiled chains of molecules which if unraveled and tied together would form a fragile string more than 6 feet long but only 50 trillionths of an inch wide. All living creatures contain at least one chromosome. Each species maintains a specific number of chromosomes per cell. Chromosome number is not necessarily related to one's physical or mental prowess; for example, human cells normally contain 46 chromosomes, cotton plants have 52, turkeys 82, and some ferns can boast of more than 1000 chromosomes per cell. Of more importance is the chemical structure of the chromosomes. The word chromosome means "colored body" and refers to nineteenth-century microscopists' observations that the chromosomes pick up the basic red or purple dyes used in nuclear stains. We now know that each chromosome is a long strand of the chemical *deoxyribonucleic acid*, known simply as DNA. Along the length of this long, unbranched molecule of DNA there are attached clusters of beadlike proteins termed histones. The DNA strand is densely coiled and forms the slightly bent rodlike body seen through the microscope. As ordinarily viewed, the chromosomes appear inert, like sticks scattered across the landscape. But they hold the deepest secrets of the cell.

For there reside the *genes*, the chromosomal subunits in which lies the code that determines a lot more than our hair and eye color, our sex, or our height, and right- or left-handedness. They are the direct cause of many diseases such as cystic fibrosis and sickle-cell anemia, regulate our tendency toward cancer, heart attacks, or Alzheimer's disease . . . in fact, humans are afflicted by more than 3000 known inherited diseases. We have identified the responsible gene for less than 3% of these. The term genome refers to all of the genetic material in the chromosomes of a particular organism.

So there is much to explain about the nature of the gene and all that it implies. But first we must look at DNA, the stuff of which genes are made.

The exciting search for the precise structure of DNA is considered to be the greatest biological saga to date in this century. In 1953 a 24-year-old American graduate student, James Watson, now a leading figure in the HGP, and Francis Crick, the English physicist turned molecular biologist, collaborated at the Cavendish Laboratory at Cambridge University to win an international race that answered this very question.

Biological systems often reveal the key to their function through their structure. Such was the result of this team's epic achievement. The uncovering of the invisible molecular structure of DNA brought the Nobel prize in 1962 to Watson, Crick, and Maurice Wilkins, the latter a colleague at King's College. And what a marvelously beautiful and symmetrical molecule it is. It functions as a deceptively simple, gently twisted chain of only four kinds of repeating units—the nucleotides. These consist of a phosphate group, the sugar deoxyribose, and a nitrogen-containing base. The difference among the four types of nucleotides resides in the nitrogenous bases. Each nucleotide contains either adenine (A), guanine (G), cytosine (C), or thymine (T). The entire molecule is shaped like an evenly twisted ladder, the sidepieces made up of alternating sugar and phosphate groups, with the rungs consisting of nitrogenous bases attached to the sugars. The rungs are actually pairs of bases loosely attached to each other. Due to the twisted nature of the DNA "ladder" only A can bind to T, and G to C.

Therein lies the answer to the mystery and power of DNA. A code is imprinted in the precise sequence of nitrogenous bases running down the length of the DNA molecule. Just as a series of numbers can program a computer to perform assigned functions, the sequence of nitrogenous bases just as certainly spells out a code that sets in place all of the cell's activities. The code consists of a series of bases, ATT, GCC, GAT, or any other combination of three out of the four nitrogenous bases. A brief calculation will quickly reveal that there are only 64 possible combinations of three bases. How can this brief code operate one cell, let alone the 100 trillion cells in an adult human?

The system works because of what these base triplets code for, that is, the making of proteins. Just as the DNA molecule is a long chain of sugar, phosphate, and nitrogenous base building blocks, proteins are long chains of units termed amino acids. There are 20 chemically different amino acids in human proteins. When attached end to end in a specific sequence and then folded up like complex pretzels, these amino acid chains form the thousands of different proteins needed by our cells. A typical protein is made up of many hundreds of amino acids.

It is easy to see how protein types can be so varied, for a single change in the position of a few or sometimes even one amino acid can change the nature of that protein. For example, a difference in one amino acid in the hemoglobin molecule causes a deficiency in its oxygen-carrying capacity. The result is the devastating disease sickle-cell anemia. Quite simply, the code in the DNA for this amino acid is scrambled and the protein produced is therefore abnormal.

Let us assume that a sequence of ATT in the DNA is the code for amino acid type 1. Let us further assume that GCC is the code for amino acid 2 and so on until we have codes for all 20 amino acids. Scientists have discovered the identity of all such codes. We now know that the sequence of nitrogenous bases in the DNA molecule determines the sequence of amino acids in the proteins made by the cell. In other words, DNA is in charge of sending a message to the cell in which it resides to make specific proteins. Why is this so important?

In addition to being used as a structural framework of the cell, a scaffolding, so to speak, on which the components of the cell are built and as an energy source, proteins control the cell's *metabolism*.

What happens in a living cell? The answer is deceptively simple— thousands of chemical reactions, otherwise known as metabolism. If one could perch on the cell membrane and watch cellular life in action, one would witness a dazzling array of rapid chemical interactions. But this would not be the chemistry of the test tube or of the laboratory bench.

This is the chemistry of life itself, a maelstrom of swirling molecules, seemingly random but upon close examination extraordinarily ordered—a self-regulating dynamic chemical sea.

That which distinguishes the chemistry of life from that of nonlife is, in a word, organization. In a living cell, chemicals—for example, hormones or sugars—are synthesized until their concentration is sensed by the cell to be correct and then their production is slowed or ceased until more are needed. In another instance, a complex molecule, no longer required, is broken down into simple molecules which are then recruited as building blocks to synthesize other cellular requirements. And so it goes as the cell, while "nothing more" than a sea of chemicals, is able to grow, maintain, repair, and even reproduce itself.

What drives these living chemical reactions? What makes them possible in the first place? They are brought about by proteins called *enzymes*. These proteins' critical importance is their ability to act as catalysts which induce molecules to combine to form new combinations or to allow the more complex molecules to break down into smaller components.

Therefore, that which makes one species of organism different from another related species, or what makes one human different from another, can be stated simply: they differ in the code carried by their DNA. That code determines which enzymes are made, and the enzymes control which chemical reactions can occur. If I have your DNA code, we are identical twins. Our chemical reactions are identical and our cells will act alike, following the directions written into the DNA. We follow the orders of DNA. We have no choice. We are prisoners of our genes.

To add to the problem, not all genes act directly upon the cell. Many genes act by influencing the activity of other genes. The job of these genes is to actually "turn on" or "turn off" other genes. Consider, for example, certain cells in the retina of the eye. They must develop into cells of a particular shape and size which make pigments—those colored chemicals which react to the incoming light and make visual reception possible. In contrast, cells in the muscles of the arm are much larger and broader, have many nuclei, and must manufacture proteins enabling them to be contractile. In both types of cells there are exactly the same number and kinds of chromosomes. Obviously, not all of the genes in these differing cell types are actually "turned on." If they were, chaos would result. In each cell, wherever it may happen to be located in the body, some genes operate and others are "turned off." Very little is understood about how this is regulated.

So finally, what actually are the genes? How do they fit into this story of life's chemistry? For our present purposes, a gene is to be considered that segment of the DNA molecule that contains the code for a particular protein. Considering the large size of most proteins, that means that a gene contains a specific sequence of thousands of nitrogenous bases. There are somewhere between 50,000 and 100,000 genes in each human cell. The genome is one complete set of these genes. It is the entire code, hidden in the genes, that the HGP seeks to discover.

The extent of the current ignorance about our genes should be immediately obvious when we must make what amounts to a wild guess about how many we actually have. To add to the problem, many scientists have concluded that less than 2% of our genes contain useful information, that is, codes that direct protein synthesis. Approximately 50 million pairs of nitrogenous bases are the blueprint of life. The remaining 98% is regarded by many to be nonfunctional, so that the chromosome may be a string of "useless" genes discarded by evolution, punctuated here and there by the message that keeps us alive.

The HGP would never have been considered possible without the existence of a series of remarkable discoveries beginning in 1970 which have drastically changed the focus and scope of biological science. These were initiated by the development of a method to remove specific segments of chromosomes using enzymes termed "restriction endonucleases" isolated from bacteria. We now have hundreds of different kinds of these enzymes which make it possible deliberately and specifically to cut up chromosomes into variously sized fragments containing genes.

This method rapidly led to the technique of combining genes from diverse sources such as bacteria, plants, or animals using the enzyme "ligase." In 1973 Stanley Cohen of Stanford University and Herbert Boyer of the University of California at San Francisco first used these procedures to insert genes from the African clawed toad into bacterial cells. The toad genes proceeded to function normally in the bacterial cells. This bizarre gene combination was in itself of no use. The toad was simply a convenient laboratory animal whose DNA was available. The enormous significance of this functional combination was that for the first time genes had combined in a unique workable mix across the barriers of millions of years of evolution separating the bacterial and animal kingdoms. A new era of hitherto unimagined control over living organisms had begun.

The rapid and widespread application of the Boyer and Cohen techniques has become familiar in the popular press as "genetic engineering." Scientists now routinely transfer human genes into simple organisms such as yeast and bacteria, converting them into useful "factories" producing valuable proteins such as insulin or the blood-clot-dissolving medication TPA (tissue plasminogen activator), both of which are now commercially available. Plans are underway for transfers of human genes into cows to trigger the manufacture of the human gene protein product in the cows' milk. The cow may become a living factory for the production of useful human gene products such as hormones.

Fanciful gene combinations can be formed, exemplified by the case in which the firefly "luciferase" genes have been introduced into carrots, creating plants which literally can be made to glow in the dark. Illuminated carrots offer no agricultural advantage, but connecting genes such as luciferase to more useful genes offers the researcher a visible sign that a successful gene introduction has been accomplished. The firefly gene acts as a "marker," causing the recipient organism to glow and signaling that the useful gene joined to it is probably there as well.

The humble yeast, by the way, a microscopic single-celled fungus, has emerged as an extraordinarily important organism in the study and implementation of modern genetics. Yeast can be grown rapidly and in great numbers in the laboratory and its hereditary characteristics can be easily followed. Also, yeast can be genetically engineered to carry very large segments of chromosomes from bacterial, plant, or animal sources in "yeast artificial chromosomes." The creature that for thousands of years has been our willing servant providing us with bread and alcohol has taken on a new and vital role.

Within a few years we have gone from the time-honored practice of interbreeding various plants as well as animals, which has been the traditional source of our modern agricultural crops and domestic livestock, to our present era. Now, at least in theory, genes from any organism can be introduced into any other organism to create novel life forms. The unlimited possibilities in the dicing and splicing of genetic combinations have spawned research and development at a dizzying pace. By the early 1980s these extraordinary developments had set the stage for the tantalizing possibility of a successful concerted attempt to map and sequence the entire human genome. A complete genome map would give the location of the genes on each of the 46 chromosomes, while a genomic sequence would be the sequence of nitrogenous bases in the nucleotides making up the DNA of those chromosomes, in other words, the genetic code.

In 1984 a small group of molecular biologists met in Alta, Utah at the invitation of the U.S. Department of Energy (DOE). The DOE had a congressional mandate to study the genetic damage inherited by the children of people who had been exposed to low levels of radiation and other mutation-causing agents. None of the assembled experts had investigative tools at their disposal with which to accomplish this on a large scale and in a reasonable period of time. These kinds of changes occur at the genetic level and would necessitate the ability to detect as few as one altered nitrogenous base out of 10 million. They knew that in order to accomplish this they would have to decipher the nitrogenous base sequence of the entire human genome.

In May 1985, Robert Sinsheimer, the chancellor of the University of California at Santa Cruz, had taken the idea of comprehensive human genome sequencing seriously enough to assemble a group of scientists on his campus in hopes that such a project, if thought to be feasible, might be centered at his university.

Others began to champion the idea, notably Renato Dulbecco of the Salk Institute in La Jolla, California. He wrote in March 1986 that sequencing the human genome would be a "turning point in cancer research." It could, according to Dulbecco, lead scientists to the genes involved in triggering malignancy. These words of a scientist of international reputation caught the attention of the scientific community.

The idea had other prominent supporters as well. Charles DeLisi, director of the DOE Office of Health and Environmental Research proposed, after a conference in Santa Fe, New Mexico in March 1986, that DOE laboratories should be the center of this effort. In fact, the discussions at Santa Fe revolved around precisely how the sequencing ought to be carried out, not whether it should be done at all. The DOE had, after all, been involved in human genetics studies for years, and had established the National Gene Library Project based at their Los Alamos and Lawrence Livermore laboratories. This "library" is a collection of human DNA fragments of known size that are freely available to researchers. Additionally, in 1983 the DOE had put together its Genbank, the major DNA sequence data bank at Lawrence Livermore.

The DOE envisioned the HGP as a natural progression of this approach albeit on a hitherto unimagined scale. Nobel laureate Walter Gilbert of Harvard University, one of the early developers of genome sequencing methods, went so far as to proclaim that "sequencing the human genome is like pursuing the holy grail."

Sparked by such flights of rhetoric, rumors that the DOE was about to undertake a large-scale human genome project had spread throughout the scientific community. To many, the very idea seemed almost ludicrous. After all, scientists knew that the genetic blueprint of a typical bacterial cell is almost 5 million nitrogenous base pairs long. For a microscopic yeast cell it is 15 million base pairs. In a human being the genetic sequence is some 3 billion base pairs. Deciphering the human genome using the then-available methodologies would have literally taken centuries.

Enter an almost legendary figure. James Watson, Nobel laureate, co-discoverer of the molecular structure of DNA and now the director of the world-renowned Cold Spring Harbor Laboratory on Long Island, New York, led the proponents of the HGP during the course of a 1986 Cold Spring Harbor symposium on the "Molecular Biology of *Homo sapiens.*" However, he voiced serious concern over the prospect of the DOE being deeply involved in what would essentially be a project in the biological sciences.

Instead he proposed that the project be centered in the National Institutes of Health (NIH). Watson pointed out that the leaders of the DOE were traditionally physical scientists for whom biology naturally occupied a lower position on their list of priorities. The NIH on the other hand is led by biologists and the NIH is the traditional funding agency for projects of a fundamentally biological nature.

Despite Watson's unquestioned stature, many other scientists at that meeting voiced serious objections. Their overriding concern, beyond the question of the administration of such an ambitious effort, which at that time was expected to bear a price tag of $2 billion, was that it would divert funding from other biological research, including projects of equal or greater merit in the eyes of many scientists. After all, the proponents of a concerted effort to sequence the human genome had to admit that they lacked efficient laboratory procedures, sufficiently trained personnel, and the computer technology necessary to make the project feasible.

But the idea had developed a life of its own. David Baltimore, a widely respected biochemist at the Whitehead Institute remarked: "The idea is gaining momentum. I shiver at the thought." Knowing that the then-current methods at hand for genome sequencing were tedious, time consuming, and labor intensive led Baltimore and others to be initially overwhelmed at the magnitude of the proposal.

The growing controversy aroused the attention of the Board of Basic Biology, Commission of Life Sciences of the National Academy of Sciences. In August 1986 they appointed a special National Research Council Committee to study the matter and make recommendations as to what ought to be done. After 14 months of deliberations the committee unanimously urged that the U.S. Congress begin the HGP and invited other nations jointly to pursue this as a common effort.

Next, the Office of Technology Assessment (OTA) of the U.S. Congress was directed by the House Committee on Energy and Commerce to prepare a report. This report would assess the scientific and medical reasons for an HGP as well as the funding mechanisms, coordination among agencies, and the posture of the United States toward cooperating with other countries while maintaining its competitive position in biotechnology. The findings were prepared with the advice and assistance of several hundred experts drawn from the fields of science, medicine, law, business, and ethics.

While the 1988 OTA report did not offer specific recommendations but rather informed Congress on the options for further action, the message of the 218-page report was quite clear. The HGP was no longer to be regarded as something whose feasibility was to be debated further but as a *fait accompli* and Congress had a vital role to play in its implementation. Within the space of 2 years what had begun as interesting speculation had snowballed into a policy of the nation's scientific community.

Actually, elements of the HGP, though not under that title, had been already underway in a piecemeal fashion. DOE and NIH both had genome study projects budgeted for 1987 to the extent of $29.2 million. Additional research was being carried out by the National Science Foundation (NSF) and by private agencies, most notably the Howard Hughes Medical Institute (HHMI). The HGP was to be a quantum leap in the scale and complexity of such efforts. In view of the multifaceted approach to human genome analysis, in its report the OTA panel noted that "there is no single human genome project, but instead many projects."

What had happened in these few years to change the concept of sequencing the human genome from what had begun as a rather nebulous and daunting concept proposed by disparate sources to a full-scale project? In 1986 Joseph Gall of the Carnegie Institution of Washington had warned, "My plea is simply that we think about this project in light of what we already know about . . . genetics and not set in motion a scientifically ill-advised Juggernaut." In 1987 Leroy Hood and Lloyd Smith at the California Institute of Technology would proclaim "the sequence of the human genome would be perhaps the most powerful tool ever developed to explore the mysteries of human development and disease." By 1990 James Watson could confidently announce in the renowned international journal *Science* that "the United States has now set as a national objective the mapping and sequencing of the human genome."

Part of the answer as to how it became a reality so quickly lies in a summary of the rapid evolution of the specific objectives of the HGP. What had first seemed like a utopian goal of determining the nitrogenous base sequence of the entire human genome had been soon modified to feature, among other related objectives, the creation of human chromosome *maps*. The goals for the period 1990–1995 had become the detailed construction of "genetic linkage maps," "physical maps," and the development of "DNA sequencing technology."

There are several new concepts involved here. Genetic linkage maps are constructed by studying families and measuring the frequency with which two different traits are inherited together, or linked. Put simply, it is analyzing the familiar "family tree" in terms of certain measurable characteristics, often by following the inheritance of a particular disease. The logic behind this approach is that if two genes or group of genes responsible for two different characteristics are located near each other on the same chromosome, the chances of them being inherited are much greater than those located far apart or on separate chromosomes.

This approach has its distinct disadvantage when applied to humans, because of the necessity to follow carefully the genetic details of extended family trees whose history extends over generations. After all, one has to wait an average of almost 20 years after the birth of an individual before he or she becomes a parent. Experimental animals such as *Drosophila* (the fruit fly) which have been studied extensively in genetics laboratories complete their life cycle from birth through reproduction to death within several weeks. The bacterium *Escherichia coli*, arguably the organism with the most intensively analyzed genome, can divide and copy itself every 20 minutes.

Physical maps, on the other hand, are derived principally from chemical analysis of the DNA molecules themselves that make up the genome. There are several different categories of physical maps but all maps share a common goal of placing the location of human genes in a linear order according to their relative position along the chromosomes. Remember the analogy of the chromosome being like a long string of beads, each bead representing a gene. If we assume that each bead has a number on it, these physical and linkage maps would give clues about the numerical sequence of the beads in the chain. Knowing the location of the genes and their corresponding genetic traits allows scientists to discover patterns of genome organization and how they correspond to important functions as well as compare humans with other mammals.

We humans share many identical genes with a host of other organisms. Although, for example, we are separated from the primates by at least 30 million years of evolution, our chromosomes differ from those of the chimpanzees in approximately 1% of the genes. Relatively few nitrogenous base messages stand between life in the trees and life in the suburbs. Precious little DNA differs between the zoo keepers and the zoo inhabitants.

Laborious research had led to the determination of large portions of the DNA sequence of relatively primitive subjects such as viruses and bacteria. Small groups of scientists had spent years in the attempt to sequence a single gene. Since the human DNA sequence is orders of magnitude larger, using this hands-on method would take centuries to decipher the entire human genome. A "cottage industry" approach involving small numbers of individuals working independently, traditionally the *modus operandi* of biologists, could never accomplish the task.

The solution had to be in technological breakthroughs, and this is precisely what had begun to occur. Automation was to be the answer to the problem of the staggering number of person-hours needed to sequence 3 billion base pairs. By 1990 the use of automated DNA sequencers had reduced the cost of sequencing to $5 per base pair and were operating at the rate of 10,000 bases per day, still too slow and too expensive but remarkably better than just a few years earlier.

However, beyond the consideration of such factors as technological advances and plans for organizational restructuring, we must come back to the crux of the rapid and enthusiastic expansion of the HGP from theory to practice. The key to this phenomenon ultimately lies in the nature of scientific inquiry and the motivation of those who engage in it as their life's work. Looking at it from their perspective, who could object to this marvelous project? The HGP had become "beautiful science."

The Manhattan Project during World War II at Los Alamos (ironically now a principal site of HGP research) where scientists harnessed atomic energy, held out to the physicists of that day the lure of unlocking the power of the atom. So too the Apollo Project, designed to propel human beings to the moon and back took on the symbolic role of national pride. The architects of that extraordinary feat were engineers who were engrossed in the technological challenge of launching a massive projectile to arc through space and land its human cargo gently on another planet. Now the prospect of an unprecedented all-out effort to decipher the very code of life held out a similar attraction for biologists.

For what motivates scientists? To be sure, the enhancement of personal reputation and financial rewards can be driving forces. More important is the satisfaction of fulfilling one's burning curiosity about how the systems around us operate. Biologists want to know how and why the birds migrate thousands of miles and return inexorably to their summer territory, how the minute egg unfolds into the multicellular adult, and how a green leaf transforms the sunlight into sweet molecules of sucrose.

To many of today's brightest scientific minds the opportunity to translate the language of DNA—the molecule that in a real sense controls all of life—into words that we can understand is irresistible.

Yet there is another aspect operative here which we must consider to complete the picture of all of those forces which motivate the scientist.

Behind the familiar generalities of "scientific curiosity" and "expanding the horizons" of our knowledge lies another principal aim of science—control.

Examples of such control are numerous. Since the diabetic pancreas can no longer regulate its own insulin production we can control the sugar level in a diabetic's blood by insulin injections because we have discovered that this chemical regulates the entrance of sugar into our cells. We control the timing of flower production in many ornamentals because we understand that the relative length of the light and dark periods triggers the flowering response in those plants. We can control pests in our trees. Biologists have gathered data on the attractiveness of gaseous hormones released by female gypsy moths. This has led to the synthesis of attractants that lure the males of the species to their deaths, sparing trees from destructive defoliation. Such examples are the obviously pragmatic fruit of scientific discoveries. Yet they pale in comparison with the control that could result from a complete understanding of the human chromosomes.

Chromosomes are not simply purveyors of our general characteristics and some diseases. They are literally made up of the molecules that control all living organisms. In the individual architecture and communal arrangement of genes within the chromosomes lie the directions for building, maintaining, and operating the complex machinery of the cell.

The sperm and egg cell form in the sexually mature human by the process of meiosis, in which cells in the male testes and female ovaries reduce their chromosome numbers (shared by the rest of the cells of the body) from 46 to 23. When fertilization occurs, the 46 are reunited and within that unique complement of genes the instructions begin to emerge within a few hours, first to create new cells and within a few days, as the young embryo nestles into the protective lining of the womb, orders to expand into the marvelously complex process of forming the human child have begun.

To truly understand the genes in both structure and function will be to gain the possibility of control over them and all that they do. And that, all rhetoric aside, is the ultimate aim of the Human Genome Project.

Let us look at an example of what this control would mean. In

August 1989, after years of persistent and painstaking searching through strands of DNA isolated from the blood and tissues of 100 families of cystic fibrosis sufferers, researchers announced that they had located the defective gene causing this devastating disease and had also isolated its protein product. Cystic fibrosis is the most common lethal inherited disease among people of Western European descent. One in 22 Caucasians carries the abnormal gene which is passed on in a recessive pattern, meaning that a person must inherit two abnormal genes, one from each parent, to be affected.

Francis S. Collins of the University of Michigan in Ann Arbor, along with colleagues Lap-Chee Tsui and John R. Riordan of the University of Toronto, found the gene on chromosome number 7. It has a 250,000 base code which contains a subtle "misspelling." Seventy percent of the time a change in just three nitrogenous bases in the gene code results in a defective protein. In other words, the gene functions perfectly normally except for the fact that it produces a protein which is missing just one amino acid called phenylalanine. This amino acid defect is enough to change the function of the protein. There are exactly 1480 amino acids in the protein. The gene is actually quite large and as is often the case is a mosaic of many separate actively coding areas interrupted by noncoding sequences.

The protein made by the gene belongs to a group of compounds that are involved in transporting salt and water across cell membranes. In cystic fibrosis, cells in the lungs, sweat glands, pancreas, and intestines show abnormal transport, so that salt and water build up outside the cells and mucus on the outside of the cells becomes thick and sticky. The abnormal mucus in the lungs traps bacteria that cause pneumonia and other infections. Many people with cystic fibrosis die before the age of 30.

Having determined the location of the abnormal gene, the normal gene can be isolated and produced in large quantities in the laboratory. The availability of large quantities of the normal gene raises the possibility of introducing this chromosome segment into patients to overcome the harmful effects of the abnormal gene. Cystic fibrosis—since its main effects are in the lungs—may even be vulnerable to treatment by inhaling a drug which would correct the faulty protein. Techniques are being devised for such attempts with this and other genes that cause different diseases.

This then stands as a classic example of how analysis of DNA and identification of a specific gene and its product promises control—that is, a potential cure or preventive measure for a devastating disease. The cystic fibrosis gene story is a prime example of what has already been accomplished in the scrutiny of the human genome and serves as a model of the scientific approach to such an important puzzle.

This discovery of a disease-causing gene and the development of a method to recognize it will permit testing of adults to determine whether they harbor the gene and whether they would be at risk of having an affected child. If their partner also carries the gene, the odds for each of their children inheriting the disease is one in four. This possibility of informing prospective parents of the health risk to their children by genetic analysis must be considered an awesome achievement. Genetic studies and consequent counseling have already become a common practice and as the knowledge of human genes progresses by leaps and bounds, as envisioned by the leaders of the HGP, a bewildering array of genes will be identifiable. The pressure to undergo such an analysis will be tremendous and couples will be faced with an unprecedented array of information about the odds of their offspring inheriting diseases or even tendencies toward diseases.

What's more, such genetic screening can, of course, be done on the developing fetus. By the removal of a few fetal cells, chromosomes can be analyzed and harmful genes easily identified. The abortion decision takes on a new dimension when parents are presented with a clear picture of what health problems their child will be facing.

Another significant question concerns the commercial aspects of a scientific search which leads to a gene. Scientists normally publish their results in scientific journals whose editorial board exercises careful scrutiny over the articles which they approve for publication. In the case of the cystic fibrosis gene story at least two dozen scientists at two institutions and a half-dozen funding agencies in two countries participated in the research. Somehow the news of the discovery was leaked to the press. This short-circuited the standard route of publication in a science journal followed by peer review. Given the enormous publicity the principal researchers consented to hold two press conferences before the scheduled publication date of their breathtaking research. Because of the publicity another element came into play. Frantic activity ensued among university and hospital officials, as they had to accelerate their preparations for filing patent applications.

Patents on a scientific discovery? Yes, for the techniques necessary to isolate and identify a particular gene are regarded much the same as an invention. After all, these techniques allow for the first time a routine screening procedure to determine if members of the general population are carrying the defective gene. In order to establish priority for a scientific achievement the date and sometimes even the exact time of day on which a written report is received by a journal is recorded. This establishes the authors of the report as owners of the discoveries related in the article.

In the case of the methodology for detecting the cystic fibrosis gene the royalties will be enormous. In this case they will be shared by the Hospital for Sick Children, the University of Michigan, and the Howard Hughes Medical Institute. Should such a discovery become the property of institutions or individuals? Will a whole array of human genes come to be "owned" by persons who will have a legal right to their use? We have entered an unprecedented era of social and ethical puzzles.

Prominent among such complex questions are the following—by no means a complete list of the many questions to be explored.

Is genetic information merely a more detailed account of a person's vital statistics, or should it be treated as private, not to be sought or disclosed without the individual's expressed consent?

Should diagnostic genetic information about disorders for which there is no cure be handled differently from that concerning disorders for which there is intervention?

What are the dangers inherent in manipulating genes in the laboratory or introducing them into humans?

What are the implications of allowing parents to determine the genetic endowment of their children?

What facets, if any, of human genome mapping and sequencing should be commercialized?

Do scientists have a duty to share information? What are the practical extent and limits of such an obligation?

Will genetic screening be a requirement for employment or insurance coverage?

What will the long-term effect of genetic diagnosis and manipulation be on how we view ourselves as human persons?

What are "good" genes and "bad" genes, and who will decide?

What ethical issues are raised when considerations of international competitiveness influence basic scientific research?

Given the possibilities for the alleviation of human suffering inherent in the mapping and sequencing of the human genome do we have a right not to do it?

We must keep in mind that in spite of the lofty ideals expressed by the acknowledged leaders of the project one must not lose sight of the fact that through this effort—pregnant with the possibilities of major discoveries throughout—reputations will be made and enhanced, Nobel prizes will be won, and personal and corporate fortunes will be made. This uncomfortable blend of pure science and entrepreneurship meet in the HGP on a major scale and is constantly reshaping the history of this intriguing search for the "holy grail" of science.

       *   *   *

Planet Earth, rotating slowly on the outer edge of its galaxy, one among uncounted billions of galaxies, congealed from a swirling mass of matter 4.6 billion years ago. As Earth cooled and the vast oceans formed from relentless rains, molecules coalesced in the warmth of the primordial chemical soup, energized by raging electrical storms. Organic molecules (those containing the carbon atom) formed temporary associations, a transient ever-changing population of nature's experiments. And then, within a billion years after the Earth's birth, primitive cells appeared. Those pale microscopic spheroids of complex organic molecules teemed in the warm shallow bays and lagoons. They were alive—no longer at the total mercy of their environment, but possessed of an awesome capacity to self-regulate, to take in chemical building blocks, to release unnecessary toxic waste products, and most importantly to reproduce. They could literally make copies of themselves. Life, once formed in the prehistoric brine, has continued, changing, evolving, and in the words of Charles Darwin that conclude *The Origin of Species*:

> There is grandeur in this view of life, with its several powers, having been originally breathed by the Creator into a few forms or into one; and that, whilst this planet has gone cycling on according to the fixed laws of gravity, from so simple a beginning endless forms most beautiful and most wonderful have been, and are being evolved.

Billions of years of evolution have resulted in many millions of species, most of which are now extinct. The living organisms on our planet now represent the tips of the branches of an enormous evolutionary tree. Only one species, an animal, going by the name of *Homo sapiens*, has developed over the last 450,000 years the ability to reason.

The ceaseless curiosity, imprinted in the primitive brain and applied over the centuries, ultimately gave rise to modern science. Out of this systematic and dogged pursuit over the last few decades, the workings of the living world have come under intense and unprecedented scrutiny. In the ultimate paradox of life born out of a dead earth, the key to the innermost control of living cells has at long last been discovered by complex aggregations of those very cells, called human beings. An organism driven by genes has discovered the biological key which enables itself to make the discovery of its own components.

Increased understanding of the genes, and the emergence of the technology to begin to study them intensively, has culminated in the Human Genome Project, a full-scale assault on what remains, in spite of all of our advances, a fascinating enigma.

Biological scientists are now collecting and analyzing data about our genes at an ever-increasing pace. They are creating a scenario in which the way we look at humans will be forever altered. What will they and we do with this power? A challenge greater than that of acquiring this knowledge may yet be ours: the wisdom to use it wisely. We hope that the succeeding pages will contribute to a deeper understanding of this fascinating and challenging story and assist in the decisions that will soon be ours to make.

2

THE FIRST SYNTHESIS

The fascinating, convoluted history of the search for explanations of the nature of heredity began with vague, unspecified notions of unseen forces directing the reproduction and development of living things. It has evolved into the current intensive, specific, and highly technical analysis of the precise function and molecular details of the gene. A simple chronological rendering of names and discoveries cannot adequately convey either the paradigmatic nature of that search within the living world or the role of scientists in helping to shape those insights.

The tale of the discovery of first the physical and then the chemical organization of the cells, the nucleus, the chromosomes, and finally that of the genes exemplifies a profound transmutation of thought and attitude in Western society. This change must be understood if one wishes to appreciate fully the forces and motives that direct such current scientific activities as the Human Genome Project.

Science as we know it is basically a product of the nineteenth and twentieth centuries. Observation, experimentation, statistical analysis, widespread communication among scientists, and objective critical evaluations of theories are comparatively recent phenomena. The discipline within the biological sciences that has undergone extraordinary development in our century and has had the most profound impact on the progress of biology as a whole has undoubtedly been genetics, the study of the mechanisms of hereditary transmission and variation of organismal characteristics. The very term genetics is new to this century. It was an invention of the English biologist William Bateson in 1905. The story of genetics, how it came to exist as a specific discipline, and its extraordinary development in our century is the story of the complex path which has led to the Human Genome Project; its rationale cannot be fully understood without a brief analysis of how modern science itself has evolved.

Humans, one must assume, have always sought to make sense of their surroundings and of themselves. The gradual change from the conviction that the sky was a dome with the heavenly bodies in fixed positions to an awakening that the universe is in constant motion has had its counterpart in the observations of and puzzlement over living organisms. All forms of life appeared to generate others of the same kind. The creatures of the land, sea, and air multiplied in great numbers. However, like always produced like. There were many individual differences among the various kinds of birds or fish or land creatures but they were always recognizable as members of a specific type which remained, as far as any observer could see, apparently consistent.

Since the dawn of agriculture some 12,000 years ago, humans have depended on what they knew of their plants' reproductive processes and have gradually manipulated their crops by intentional matings of varieties to produce plants that, though mostly similar, had measurably new and useful characteristics. Our modern-day agricultural crops, upon which the life of humanity has come to depend, are a result of deliberate crossbreedings and selection of the most desirable offspring for further propagation. Even before the scientific genetic basis for these manipulations was known, humans used their empirical insights to improve edible plants and domesticated animals as well.

Our human species, *Homo sapiens*, has existed on earth for approximately 450,000 years of earth's almost 5-billion-year history. For all but the last several centuries almost all of the workings of the world, both living and inanimate, have been complete and utter mysteries. The unfathomable rising of the sun, the dawning of spring, the annual migration and reappearance of the birds, the beating of our hearts, and the striking similarity between child and parent despite their unique features necessitated elaborate tales to offer some satisfactory explanations.

These rationales often have been embodied in a rich complex of myths, art, and customs. Gradually individuals with particular curiosity and the courage to question the simplistic yet almost instinctive explanations of natural phenomena began to study them in a more systematic way. Their logically acceptable explanations began to replace myth with reality. The ancient Greeks were the first culture to undertake what we would consider organized scientific inquiry and to seek explanations of the universe and of themselves in a deeper way.

They developed the basic elements of mathematics, astronomy, physics, geography, and medicine. However, what we know as the biological sciences, the study of living organisms, can truly be said to have begun in a productive sense only in the seventeenth century as early microscopists began to peer into details of microbial and cellular life. Even so, it was not until the nineteenth century that there developed, at first tentatively, with a few conflicting observations and experiments, and then in a burst of discoveries and theories toward the latter part of the century, an impetus that catapulted biological science onto a trajectory which has led to our current understanding of the intricacies of living systems and thereby the development of modern science, medicine, and agriculture.

The reasons behind the sudden flowering of science within the lifetime of only a few generations have to do in part with a transition which was not strictly scientific but also philosophical. It was based on a radical change from addressing all phenomena through answers derived from religion and philosophy to an objective scrutiny marked by close, systematic observation and careful repeated experimentation. Deeper than simply a methodological shift, the approach was sustained by a worldview that has been described as *mechanism*, as opposed to *vitalism*. While all historical generalities are imperfect, this distinction is a clear one. It is necessary to make it here to emphasize and clarify how modern science operates.

Vitalism in its strict sense holds that there is a unique "life principle," a specific quality or essence that distinguishes living from nonliving objects. There is postulated some kind of nonmaterial force or spirit that regulates the material aspects of living organisms. A mechanistic worldview would hold that living creatures differ from nonliving structures only by virtue of their organization. Given the correct arrangement of specific interacting parts (which we now call molecules), life must exist. Life is not somehow greater than the sum of its parts.

The so-called life principle of vitalism has had many names, from Aristotle's "psyche" through the eighteenth-century "anima sensitiva" or "vis essentialis" to the twentieth-century's "élan vital" of Henri Bergson. All have been built upon mixtures of religious belief and assumptions of purposiveness in the actions of organisms, and were chiefly buttressed by almost total ignorance of any details of the chemical or physical functions of such organisms. This ignorance in turn supported an acceptance of vitalism. A strict adherence to vitalistic principles understandably tended to retard objective study of life systems.

From our perspective one can easily be critical of the imposition of such teleological motivations used to explain the actions of living things. We are the heirs to an extraordinary array of relatively recent discoveries about life functions—discoveries which have led to the Human Genome Project. Note that mechanism and vitalism can be viewed either as belief systems, encompassing all of one's attitudes toward life, or particularly in the case of mechanism, as simply a working model with which to view life for the pragmatic purpose of fruitful investigation.

The latter is an apt description of the day-to-day parameters within which the modern scientist operates. Regardless of one's religious convictions or lack of them, scientists have concluded that they must proceed as though mechanism is the only answer, simply because no other approach has proven as productive as this one. It has been the rigorous application of mechanistic reductionist principles which has permitted us to conquer smallpox, cholera, tuberculosis, and tetanus, to regulate the electrical system of the heart, or to probe the message of the chromosomes. Scientists are often criticized for analyzing and discussing living systems as though they were subject only to the laws of chemistry and physics. But this approach has improved and saved human life.

Critics unfamiliar with this objective, mechanistic approach may feel uncomfortable, particularly when it is applied to our own species. For example, when scientists speak of seeking the code within our genes as a key to analyzing how humans function they do not do so with the intention of denying what are deep mysteries such as the source of creativity, the sense of justice, or the stirrings of love. They are simply working in the mechanistic tradition which has answered more crucial and highly significant questions in the last hundred years than any other system of analysis in all of human history.

An early champion of the mechanistic school in this country was Jacques Loeb, author of *The Mechanistic Concept of Life*. In 1897 Loeb was an instructor of physiology at the Marine Biological Laboratory in Woods Hole, Massachusetts. He would soon be the first to induce parthenogenesis, the development of an unfertilized egg without the aid of a male sex cell, by forming fatherless sea urchins as a result of chemical stimulation. Writing to the physiologist William James, brother of the novelist Henry James, Loeb said, "Whatever appears to us as innervation, sensations, psychic phenomena, as they are called, I seek to conceive through reducing them . . . to the molecular atomic structure of the protoplasm . . ." In 1890 he wrote to Ernest Mach: "The idea is now hovering before me that man himself can act as creator even in the living nature, forming it eventually according to his will." How prescient he was, for now we have begun to do just that with our direct manipulation of genes in biotechnology. Genes are being recombined almost at will even despite the interkingdom barriers between plants and animals as well as those between humans and other animals. Firefly genes have been placed into carrots and cancer-causing genes into yeast. The rapidly increasing knowledge about our human genes is leading to our control of what has always been, until recently, out of our reach, creating endless possibilities.

Interestingly enough, some incisive comments on this mechanistic approach would be made by a young student in the building next to where Jacques Loeb was teaching and experimenting in 1897. Her name was Gertrude Stein. Later, in Paris, she would analyze the relationships between words as closely as others would study molecular interactions and her writings would change the way we hear our language. But at this time she was working closely with one of his colleagues, Franklin Pierce Mall in her course in embryology. Years later, in 1935, she would say in *Lectures in America* that "Science is continuously living with the complete description of something with ultimately the complete description of anything with ultimately the complete description of everything."

She was absolutely correct. The ultimate complete description of everything is encouraged and allowed by the mechanistic approach. It has guided scientists from atheists or agnostics to theists of all denominations and traditions. It is the attitude which has proven to be effective and upon whose fruits the modern world has come to depend. In *The Molecular Biology of the Gene* (1967), James Watson, now the director of the National Center for Human Genome Research at the National Institutes of Health, wrote "[We] have complete confidence that future research, of the intensity recently given to genetics, will eventually provide man with the ability to describe with completeness the essential features that constitute life."

Again, this might sound galling to someone not familiar with the prevailing attitudes of the scientific community. To scientists it is a quite logical and natural point of view which mirrors their commitment to the efficacy of the mechanistic approach. There is a direct analogy here with mechanistic views of nonliving systems as well. From Galileo to Newton to Einstein to Fermi there has evolved the view of matter itself as being explicable by its molecular, atomic, and finally its subatomic properties. The distinction between studies of living and nonliving are not absolute. François Jacob wrote in *The Logic of Life* (1973), "The aim of molecular biology is to interpret the properties of the organisms by the structure of its constituent molecules."

The rules of science as it is now practiced are understood by all participants. The rules are rigorous and hold one to high standards of honesty. They begin by announcing that nothing is to be held as absolutely true. A scientist does not say, "proposition x is true." He or she says, "The evidence appears to indicate that proposition x is the most logical explanation for the data as we interpret them." This leaves one always open to the possibility that new data will afford a new explanation. It is critical to understand this mind-set. Where science is concerned, the scientist is constrained not to "believe" anything. Data are collected and conclusions are reached which must always to some degree remain tentative.

When a scientist completes a research project he or she is expected to publish the results. Qualified colleagues judge the results based upon their findings, their attempts to repeat the experiments, and their own insights into the correct interpretations of the data. Only by passing through this gauntlet will the conclusions reach the status of acceptance.

The acceptance is always conditional against the day when new information may contradict the old.

There is an apocryphal story of a teacher who read to her class a letter—purportedly from President Truman—officially condemning the prevailing Soviet ideas on genetics as a perversion of scientific truth and endorsing the chromosome theory as correct. The class responded by loudly applauding the endorsement. They quickly received a fundamental lesson in the philosophy of science for the enthusiasm that they had displayed over this false report. The teacher explained that scientific theories are not "officially endorsed," regardless of the status of the endorser. Rather, theories are used as tools until deeper understandings prevail.

These then are some of the attitudes which have motivated us, the most recent descendants of those arboreal creatures who, 30 million years ago, diverged from the evolutionary path that would lead to the apes and took, to paraphrase Robert Frost, "the one less traveled by." Humans, by virtue of the evolution of our cerebral capabilities, could reach a point merely within the lifetime of our great-grandparents where one of us could turn and look back at those thousands of centuries of development. He would then begin to see, dimly but with unprecedented insight, the existence of that hitherto undiscovered evolutionary history ". . . and that has made all the difference." His name was Charles Darwin.

In 1859, an "abstract" was published detailing certain findings and theories concerning the "descent with modification" of living organisms. It was called *On the Origin of Species* by Charles Robert Darwin. His thesis was simple and buttressed by 27 years of observation and experimentation. He boldly stated that living organisms have changed gradually from simple organisms over the course of time, resulting in the complexity of forms which we now see and many others which have become extinct. They did so because of the following principles. All organisms vary one from the other and these variations are to some degree inherited. Since all organisms produce more offspring than survive to become adults, among the survivors will be those that may have inherited variations that have facilitated their adaptation to their local environment.

This *natural selection* results in a population with altered characteristics. This may eventually result in the appearance of a new species, that is, organisms which differ enough from their closest relatives so that they can no longer interbreed with them. This reproductive isolation creates differing populations of organisms which then proceed by their own variation acted upon by natural selection to generate even newer species.

As a simple example of the principle of natural selection consider animals with fur that blends into the natural background, making them less likely to be seen by predators or prey. The color of the fur is determined by the genes. Because this characteristic will assist in their survival, as compared to more conspicuous members of the same species, the camouflaged appearance will be passed on to the next generation proportionally more than the more vulnerable coloration.

Darwin's finches are a classic example of natural selection. Darwin found 13 distinct species of these birds on the Galápagos, a small cluster of islands off the west coast of South America. Apparently, after a pair of finches had been storm-blown to the remote islands from the mainland, chance variations in their descendants' beak shapes enabled some to adapt to using different types of food sources. Eventually, this separation into different habitats, such as the ground, shrubs, or forests at higher elevations, resulted in forms which differed in other ways as well, including loss of interbreeding.

The book sold out its original printing before the official publication date of November 24, 1859. It was followed by five more editions in Darwin's lifetime. It changed the course not only of biology but of human history. In the two decades that followed, his theories virtually displaced the biblical notion of a specific, divine creation of all species. His ideas resulted in a cataclysmic reversal in our understanding of the natural world.

How could a single book written by a quiet, unassuming 50-year-old biologist in failing health, living with his family in the quiet English town of Downe, have had such an extraordinary effect? And what has this episode to do with the search for the gene?

Darwin's thesis catalyzed and accelerated a transition already under way. His painstaking research and years of documented observation combined with his brilliant insights into nature crystallized the growing body of evidence for evolution and confirmed the nagging doubts that had begun to appear in the scientific community of the previous generation. For example, geology had long been considered the handmaiden of theology, and its findings had been used as evidence for phenomena such as the biblical flood. However, before the end of the eighteenth century, geologists began to uncover evidence that the earth was a great deal older than the popular estimate of a few thousand years. In *Theory of the Earth* published in 1785, James Hutton denied that a special divine force had molded the earth but that it had been and continued to be slowly transformed by natural agents such as wind, water, and subterranean movements.

Later, other geologists such as William Smith and Charles Lyell discovered rock strata bearing fossils of extinct animals, amassing evidence that species do in fact change over the ages. Even Darwin's grandfather Erasmus, who was considered an eccentric radical free-thinker, wrote the book *Zoomania* in 1794 in which he postulated that one species may change into another. In 1809, the year of Charles Darwin's birth, the French biologist Jean Baptiste de Lamarck presented his thesis, much later proven to be incorrect, that bodily characteristics acquired as the result of use or disuse of various parts or organs could be transmitted to the offspring. In this way the accumulation of such modifications could change one species into another.

In other words, he held that, to use the famous example, ancestors of giraffes must have had shorter necks, and in stretching out for leaves on higher branches extended the length of their necks ever so slightly. This increase in neck length was then inherited by the offspring. We now understand that such "acquired" charcteristics cannot be inherited because the changes have occurred in cells of the body other than the reproductive cells. Given the lack of understanding of such basic princi-ples in the nineteenth century, it was difficult to refute Lamarck's assertions.

Evolutionary ideas were "in the air." In England, that air was being visibly blackened by the expanding industrial revolution which was changing society as irreversibly as Darwin's notions were changing the world of ideas. His poor health had forced him to move with his wife from London to Downe, Kent in 1847. Left behind was a city teeming with urban poor. One of those poor, an exile from the continent, struck by the hardships suffered by the working class, was to write another book, quite different from Darwin's but equally powerful as a tool of social revolution. Karl Marx's *Das Kapital* was published in 1867.

The transition occurring in the natural sciences as well as society amplified the effects of Darwin's radical departure from the comfortable past. Science was termed "natural philosophy" before 1850, and although widespread studies of nature had been carried on with increasing interest for many years, the world was generally considered as an expression of God's creative power, goodness, and continuing care. Unfettered investigation like Darwin's into natural phenomena could not help but call into question this fundamentalist scriptural interpretation of the planet's inhabitants.

Darwin had begun his career as an amateur, an avid collector of local beetles and plants. But by the time he disembarked from the H.M.S. *Beagle* at Falmouth in October 1836 after his five-year circumnavigation as the ship's naturalist, his collection had become filled with thousands of exotic tropical creatures. These creatures made up the evidence that would gradually convince him that the variability among both plants and animals and their adaptations to their environments was a fit subject for scientific study.

He concluded that the changing and varied forms of living organisms were not, as in the best traditions of vitalism, the manifestation of a divinely guided design. The process of natural selection was a random, accidental, and therefore unplanned perpetuation of those organisms which happened to have the characteristics for survival and reproduction. This conclusion was the result of a difficult and intimidating process. In 1844 Darwin wrote to a botanist friend, Joseph Hooker, "I am almost convinced . . . that species are not (it is like confessing a murder) immutable."

In other words, Darwin was saying that the evidence did not point to a Divine Being creating all known species, which then remained forever unchanged. Rather, it indicated that those currently existing had evolved from other often simpler forms through change and natural selection operating on the results of those changes. That did not preclude the possibility of a Divine Being who was responsible for existence itself, but it certainly conflicted sharply with the literal interpretation of the scriptural creation story so widely held by Darwin's contemporaries.

In the face of growing support for Darwin's theories his opponents counterattacked with powerful arguments. Their attacks, though in many cases fueled by religious objections, were directed at Darwin's science and not his theology. The problem lay in the paucity of satisfactory explanations available for variability among organisms and the means by which these differences could be passed on to the next generation; in other words, explanations which we now call the study of heredity.

To Darwin's distress, he could draw on no adequate explanations for the source of variability among organisms. For example, why were the finches on the Galápagos closely related yet so obviously different in some of their characteristics? He felt keenly the absence of a satisfactory explanation for this obvious variability among living creatures and for its passage from one generation to the next. He was forced to accept, albeit uneasily, the explanation of Lamarck and held that characteristics acquired during a lifetime would be passed on to the offspring and thereby bring about variation within a population.

He contrived a scenario involving a provisional hypothesis whereby invisible particles which he called "gemmules" resided in all of the cells of organisms. These gemmules could be altered by environmental factors, and the sexual reproductive cells—the sperm and the egg—were composites of these modified particles. When these combined in sexual reproduction, the result was an organism with new traits that could be acted on by natural selection.

Darwin performed numerous breeding experiments in an attempt to explain variation and its inheritance. His subjects were often unfortunate choices, such as pigeons whose matings merely seemed to reinforce the single respectable theory of his time, for example, the opinion that the measurable characteristics such as the color and size of the parents sometimes blended together to appear as an unpredictable mixture in the young. If, in fact, this kind of blending inheritance was operative, then it was obvious, that differences that arose would quickly be diluted and blended away in a population. Blending could hardly be a fit subject for a selection process.

Darwin's years of painstaking effort to elucidate the source of hereditary variations were fruitless. He died on April 19, 1882, never knowing that diverse discoveries made by other scientists during his lifetime held the key to the puzzle of inheritance. But by the time of his death 23 years after the appearance of *On the Origin of Species,* this and his many other writings had gained him worldwide respect. He was laid to rest in Westminster Abbey close to Isaac Newton. It would not be until the next century that Darwin would be truly vindicated. But he had changed the world. Darwin's work had brought about, in the words of John Green, author of a 1959 book on evolution and its impact on Western thought, the "death of Adam."

A literal interpretation of Scripture could no longer be an intellectually honest or satisfying approach to the questions posed by scientific scrutiny. For many of our modern-day theologians this transition is seen as one which brought maturity to their discipline. But one needs only to follow the ongoing creationist controversy in our schools to realize how the principles of evolution, which have come to be the unifying theme of all biological investigations, are still so misunderstood and resisted by so many.

*   *   *

> It requires indeed some courage to undertake a labor of such far-reaching extent; this appears, though, to be the only right way by which we can finally reach the solution to a question the importance of which cannot be overestimated in connection with the history of the evolution of organic forms.

These are not, as one might suspect, the words of Charles Darwin. They were written in 1854, five years before the publication of *On the Origin of Species* by a contemporary of Darwin who lived in relative obscurity as a monk of the Augustinian order in a monastery in Brünn, Austria (now Brno, Czechoslovakia). The labor to which he referred was unique and elegantly simple in its conception. They are the words of Gregor Johann Mendel, whose systematic breeding experiments with peas and beans in a small monastery garden plot would uncover the fundamental laws of inheritance. His work is considered one of the greatest intellectual accomplishments in the history of science.

Johann Mendel was born in 1822 to peasant parents in the Austrian hamlet of Heitzendorf—a village that had long supplied skilled gardeners to affluent landowners. He entered the novitiate at the Abbey of St. Thomas at the age of 21 and assumed the new name of Gregor. As the Augustinians were required to supply teachers for the local secondary school, he was sent to the University of Vienna to pursue studies in the sciences and mathematics. He studied under several well-known professors of the day and, fortunately for his future studies, was introduced to the then-infant science of statistics. He returned to become a teacher of natural science and physics and lived as a monk until his death in 1884. Fortunately, the abbot of St. Thomas, F. C. Napp, had already established a busy program of plant experimentation in the monastery gardens which soon became Mendel's domain.

Mendel's methodical and meticulous experiments were quite unlike anything that had been done before. True, he was heir to a long tradition of plant breeding. Artificial fertilization of the blossoms of the date palm with pollen from the male tree was practiced in Babylonian times, although strict empirical knowledge of sexual reproduction in plants was unknown until 1694, when R. J. Camerarius demonstrated in Germany that pollen was the male character and the seed-bearing flower the female.

Another German, Joseph Köhlreuter, is considered the founder of systematic plant breeding and the direct scientific ancestor of Mendel. In 1760 he produced the first documented plant hybrid resulting from an experiment, a variety of tobacco. His pioneering work seems to have had little immediate influence on his contemporaries or immediate successors, but by the nineteenth century, serious and extensive work on plant hybridization commenced in England, France, and Germany. Thousands of experimental hybridizations were done and a wide spectrum of variability of such aspects as color, size, and shape was noted. Darwin himself made numerous crosses with flowers such as snapdragons and carefully recorded his results through several generations.

So for nearly a century, observations had been made which had the potential for yielding the principles of heredity. Only in the mind of Mendel did the grand synthesis finally occur and his story leads us a step closer to the gene.

Mendel was the first mathematical biologist. His academic training in Vienna coupled with his knowledge of and love for his plants forged a fruitful combination. Unlike any of his predecessors or contemporaries he set out to arrange in a statistically accurate way the results of deliberate crosses between varieties of pea plants with characteristics that could be clearly identified. Some have attributed his choice of peas as fortuitous but Mendel was far too careful and knowledgeable to depend on seren-dipity.

First of all, the pea is self-pollinating—that is, its delicate petals clasp and enclose the reproductive organs so that the golden pollen grains are trapped and can interact with only the female parts of the very same flower. Pea plants reproducing in this cloistered fashion will ordinarily exhibit the same physical appearance generation after generation, which is described as "true breeding." One can therefore deliberately cross plants under controlled conditions by opening the flowers early in their growth and removing the anthers, the sacs containing the then-immature pollen. Using a fine brush one can then transfer pollen from a ripe flower of another plant, a delicate and laborious task.

Mendel gathered 34 strains of pea plants from nurseries throughout Europe and spent several years carefully narrowing down his choices until he settled upon true breeding plants which differed from each other in seven pairs of traits including seed and pod form, seed color, length of stem, and position of flowers. His systematic experimental approach was novel for his time. With our hindsight derived from having been raised in an era of experimental science, Mendel's methods seem quite straightfor-ward and logical. In the 1850s he was literally at the frontiers of science with little to depend upon but his own innate sense of rigorous logic and creativity.

In a cross between plants grown from green seeds and those grown from yellow seeds, the offspring did not show a blending of these colors but were all yellow. The green trait had seemingly disappeared. Mendel then crossed members of this first yellow-seeded generation among themselves. Green seeds reappeared along with yellow seeds. But that was not all. Yellow- and green-seeded plants were formed in a specific ratio of 3:1. Mendel knew that statistical analysis was impossible without adequate numbers of plants. In a typical experiment such as the one just described we read from Mendel's accounts that he had raised and tallied

8023 hybrids! And of those, 6022 were yellow-seeded and 2001 were green.

Mendel termed the yellow trait that appeared in the first generation "dominant" and the green trait that was masked by it the "recessive." The recessive green trait had not been lost but had reappeared in what turned out to be in predictable and repeatable numbers with the next generation.

Mendel's analysis was as follows. Each trait such as seed color must be controlled by invisible *factors*, or in his original term, "elemente." Each plant would have two of these factors, having received one from each parent. There were two possible factors, a dominant one which he symbolized as A and a recessive, characterized as a. The dominant A factor would always express itself as a visible trait, in this case yellow seed color, whether present in the pair AA or Aa. The recessive a would only express itself when in combination with another, as in the combination aa.

In this specific instance, the true-breeding parent plant bearing yellow seeds would contain two dominant factors, or AA, while the true-breeding green seeded would contain two recessive, aa. Now came the critical step. In the formation of the reproductive cells (later called gametes) the pollen grain would receive only one of those factors and the female egg would likewise receive only one. Which one they received would be entirely random. In the case of a true-breeding plant such as AA or aa, only gametes with A or a were possible. If pollen bearing an A factor was crossed with eggs bearing an a factor, the resultant seeds would contain a factor combination of Aa and appear yellow. The crossing of gametes of the plants bearing either A or a in the pollen and egg yield either AA, Aa, aA, or aa. Because of the dominant nature of the A factor this would result in a 3:1 yellow to green ratio.

Mendel's next step was to consider two characteristics at a time. He crossed true-breeding plants that bore round yellow seeds with others that produced wrinkled green seeds. The first-generation seeds were all round and yellow. We can symbolize this as RRYY × rryy, which yielded RrYy. The second generation arising from crossing RrYy with RrYy yielded round yellow, round green, wrinkled yellow, and wrinkled green in a ratio of 9:3:3:1, a ratio now as familiar to the genetics student as $E = mc^2$ is to the physicist.

parents	AA (yellow) aa (green)
gametes	A x a
F$_1$	all Aa (yellow)
F$_1$ gametes	A or a x A or a
F$_2$	AA (yellow), Aa (yellow) aA (yellow), aa (green)

3:1

Each parent donates one "factor." Each offspring therefore has two. The combination of "factors" determines, in this case, the seed color, which occurs in a predictable ratio.

Mendel correctly drew several conclusions from these and many other experiments too numerous to describe here, calling them his "laws discovered for peas." The first was that one member of each pair of factors was segregated into different gametes. The chance recombination of the factors in the process of fertilization would result in plants expressing their characteristics as a function of the particular pairs of factors that they had inherited. Also, when looking at several different characteristics together such as seed color as well as shape, the factors governing these separated or "segregated" independently from each other during gamete formation.

In 1865 Mendel presented the results of eight years of research at a meeting of the Brünn Natural Science Society to an audience of local science buffs. The minutes of the meeting which, amazingly, still exist record that not a single question was asked. The listeners quickly launched into a discussion of the "hot" topic of the day—Darwin's *On the Origin of Species* which had been published six years earlier. Mendel's paper was published in the Society's journal the following year and a one-page account of his work appeared in a German encyclopedia of plant breeding. There followed, in the words of L. C. Dunn, "one of the strangest silences in the history of biology."

He sent his paper to many well-known scientists. Only the famed

German botanist Karl von Naegeli replied. He suggested that Mendel try his breeding techniques with hawkweed, one of Naegeli's favorite experimental plants, to see if the breeding of that common plant would confirm his pea results. Mendel humbly set out to follow the advice of the eminent Naegeli. He spent five frustrating years which diverted him from his other studies and ruined his eyesight. The hawkweeds showed "a behavior exactly opposite to that of peas." It was not known until 45 years later that this intractable weed often produces seeds by apogamy, that is, by development without fertilization so that crossbred offspring are sometimes, but not always, formed. This deep disappointment foreshadowed the end of Mendel's scientific work. In 1868 he was elected abbot of his monastery. His increasing administrative responsibilities until his death in 1884 put an end to his experiments.

We now know that the studious monk, by careful and insightful experimental design, had discovered the phenomenon now familiar to every introductory biology study of our day: the separation of chromosome pairs and their random distribution into gametes during the process of meiosis. Meiosis is the series of cell divisions which results in the formation of the male or female sex cells. Those are the pollen and the eggs, in the case of the flowering plants, and sperm and eggs, in the case of animals including humans.

Mendel's factors were the genes which reside in the chromosomes. The final proof of their existence, segregation during gamete production and recombination during fertilization, would have to wait until the next century, long after Mendel's death. His paradoxically fortuitous but novel insistence on mathematical analysis combined with his native modesty and reticence contributed to his lack of recognition. His goal had been to see whether there was "a generally applicable law governing the formation of the development of hybrids." He did so, but over 30 years would pass before the significance of his work was recognized.

Historians have repeatedly speculated on the effect that an application of Mendelian principles would have had on Charles Darwin's defense of his theory of evolution. The usual scenario suggests that Darwin would have been spared years of agony and indecision in reluctantly assuming the popular but incorrect blending theory of inheritance. Instead, he would have concluded that "factors"(genes) governed the expression of

physical characteristics which were randomly segregated into the reproductive cells and then recombined in the passage to the new generation.

There is no evidence that Darwin ever read Mendel's work. On the
other hand, Mendel was quite familiar with Darwin's writings as any
active scientist of the time would have been. Did Mendel see how his own
insights could buttress the evidence for the evolution of living organisms?
Did he prefer not to assist in the ascendancy of a scientific position that
appeared to oppose his religious traditions? The worlds of the staid
Victorian Englishman, father of ten children and that of the Catholic
monk, father to his monastic brethren, were farther apart than the few
hundred kilometers between the countrysides of England and Austria.

In the late seventeenth century microscopic studies with the imperfect instruments then available began to give rise to conflicting ideas
about heredity and reproduction. These studies stood in contrast to much
earlier notions of human reproduction. The ancient Greeks had thought
that infants were conceived by "coagulation" of the sperm and the
menstrual fluid. The ability of these fluids to transmit characteristics of
the parents was, according to Hippocrates, due to the fact that they
contained the "gonos" or "seed" contributed by all parts of the body
which blended to produce the child. Aristotle suggested that invisible
particles or "pangenes" came together from the body to form the
reproductive fluids. This theory of pangenesis in the best tradition of
ignorance and appeal to authority was the one preferred by both Lamarck
and Darwin 21 centuries later.

Early microscopists could not see such particles, but some, in
particular the followers of the great Dutch lens maker Anton van
Leeuwenhoek in the late seventeenth century, claimed that they could see
in each human sperm a miniature person, the "homunculus." They held
that the mother merely served as an incubator for the tiny person. During
the same period another Dutchman, Regnier de Graaf, described the
minute person as residing instead in the human egg.

While the use of primitive lenses provoked such flights of fancy, the
microscope proved to be a crucial tool in the path leading to the gene.
Robert Hooke, brilliant inventor and author of *Micrographia*, a masterful
compendium of illustrations of his microscopic studies, introduced the

term "cell" in 1665 to describe the pores that he observed in thin slices of cork tissue. Despite Hooke's impressive work the imperfect lenses in the early microscopes seriously limited their productive use for many years until the nineteenth century when major improvements were made in the lens systems by Joseph Lister, Giovanni Amici, and Ernst Abbe.

Intense interest during the last half of the nineteenth century in analyzing the actual process of reproduction was of course stimulated by the publication of *On the Origin of Species* in 1859. Three major avenues of inquiry developed: those dealing with the nature of species differences and attempts at hybridization in domesticated plants; those having to do with the details of cells, body structure, and embryological development; and others specifically concerned with the transmission of characteristics from one generation to the next. Because these investigations were driven by their reference to evolution, it is understandable that the emphasis tended to be on their application to problems of variation, evolution, and development. Research tends to be driven by the attempt to answer specific questions and such specificity would quickly develop as new information began to coalesce into a still puzzling but progressively more coherent picture. Here we briefly sketch that progression during the remarkably productive period between 1859 and 1900.

Charles Darwin, an affable man, would often spend Sunday mornings in his study or garden engaged in lively conversation with a close friend, the renowned botanist Robert Brown. According to Darwin's accounts, though Brown was of a quiet and reticent nature their conversations ranged over a wide variety of subjects. Perhaps they may have touched on Brown's report in 1831 that stated, while studying orchid leaves "in each cell . . . a singular circular areola is observable. This areola, or "nucleus" of the cell as it may be termed . . . is equally manifest among other . . . families . . ." Brown had established the nucleus as an essential part of the living cell and had named, without realizing it, the repository of the chromosomes and genes. Cytology, the study of cells, had come of age with Brown and his contemporaries and its practitioners were to play a major role in our story.

Matthias Jakob Schleiden, impressed by Brown's insights into the nucleus, formulated a new concept of the cell and its origins. He stated in

1838 that "all plants are aggregates of fully individualized, independent separate beings, namely the cells themselves." The growth of the plant, according to the German botanist, was due to the production of new cells and their subsequent development. His idea that these new cells were formed by "crystallization" around the nucleus was wrong but it brought more critical attention to bear on this puzzling structure. Equal to his contributions to the study of the cell and nucleus was his inside influence in this critical period when science was emerging from a stage of simple description and classification to one of an attempted synthesis of structure and function. He scorned a dogmatic approach, discarded the still-prevalent teleology of vitalism, and emphasized the inductive method so familiar to modern science—that is, the development of general principles from the careful study of many individual instances.

A fellow German physician and scientist, Theodore Schwann, was likewise influential in this regard. Like many others of his time he had studied under the renowned physiologist Johannes Müller, a convinced vitalist. Though a practicing Catholic, Schwann took the opposite view and adopted an extremely mechanistic and ultimately productive approach. In 1839, he published documentation that all living things were composed of cells, by which he meant the nucleus and the "layer" around the nucleus covered by a membrane. Earlier, in 1836, he had come to the extraordinarily insightful conclusion that alcoholic fermentation, decidedly a complex chemical process, was due to the metabolism of yeast, a single-celled living organism. He was vehemently attacked by the leading chemists of his day for this "heretical" suggestion. They could not accept the notion that living systems were in fact chemical sytems. This concept of life functions as chemistry would bring fame to Louis Pasteur more than 20 years later.

Schwann's description of living systems as organized bodies not produced by some vague power for a particular purpose but which evolved according to laws of necessity inherent in the properties of matter itself was a powerful and productive statement in nineteenth-century science. And yet, in keeping with the often pragmatic notion of the mechanistic approach, he could say that "I have always preferred to seek in the Creator rather than the created the cause of the finality to which the whole of nature . . . bears witness evidently." In the last years of his life he returned to the God of his earlier years, the "God of his heart, not of reason."

Schleiden and Schwann are given joint credit for establishing the cell as the common structural principle of living organisms. The emerging view of life, as nucleated units somehow functioning individually and cooperatively to produce the myriad form and function of living organisms, focused attention on these cells. By the nineteenth century, chemistry had become a highly developed science. Chemists were aware that the proportions within matter were important, for example, that "two particles of hydrogen and one particle of oxygen" combined to make water. The concept of molecules as precise amounts of elementary particles in definite relationships was clear. In 1871 in a stroke of genius, the Russian chemist Dmitri Mendeleyev arranged groups of elements in the order of their atomic weights and created the periodic table which correctly predicted the existence of several elements "missing" from this series of ascending atomic weights years before their eventual discovery.

In 1869 the Swiss chemist Johann Friedrich Meischer had isolated masses of nuclei from white blood cells by breaking down the cell membrane with digestive enzymes. The cells, gathered from pus-soaked bandages from the local hospital, yielded almost pure samples of nuclear material from which Meischer extracted high concentrations of a peculiar phosphorous-rich material which he labeled "nuclein." He surmised that the synthesis of nuclein might be a way for the cell to store phosphorous or perhaps have "something to do with heredity." By 1889 other chemists had further purified this nuclein, by removing the last traces of protein, into a gummy acidic substance, "nucleic acid." Incredibly, DNA had been isolated and purified. The bottle of innocent white powder was put away on the laboratory shelf. It would be 60 years before it would be revealed to be, in fact, what it was, a bottle of genes.

The next series of major advances would again be made with the aid of the microscope. After years of studying what might seem to be unlikely candidates for fame—the intricacies of worm cells—Friedrich Schneider, another of the many students of Johannes Müller, came upon a puzzling phenomenon. Viewing preserved and stained cells of *Mesostomium*, a transparent flatworm, Schneider saw a series of stages of the actual division of some of these cells and noted that these divisions involved a movement and separation of threadlike bodies in the nucleus. In 1873 he published a series of beautifully detailed drawings of the process. The same phenomenon was described in 1875 by Edward Strasburger who followed it within the cells of developing conifer embryos. The occurrence of this division phenomenon in both kingdoms suggested to him the possibility of the common evolutionary origin of plants and animals.

That same year the German embryologist Oskar Hertwig was the first to see a phenomenon which would lead to a critical synthesis. On a research trip to the Mediterranean he had discovered that the local sea urchins were an excellent source of abundant gametes. He returned some to his laboratory, mixed and stained the gametes, and saw that the sperm nucleus and the egg nucleus actually fused in the process of fertilization.

A few years later in 1879 an extensive survey by Walther Flemming confirmed the apparent universality of the cell division process and he named it "mitosis." He reported that as the division stages progressed, what appeared to be a continuous skein of looped threads, a "chromatin" in the nuclear area, went through a longitudinal splitting and then separated into fragments which migrated to the two resultant cells. In his studies, Flemming was the first to see human chromosomes.

Only four years later, Wilhelm Roux, in his study of the early development of frog eggs, interpreted his view of the nucleus during mitosis as a complex of macromolecules or "hereditary particles." These were parceled out to the subdividing cells as groups of particles with qualities enabling each cell to develop in ways different from the adjoining cells. He was incorrect about qualitative differences among the products of nuclear division but had managed to focus further attention on these puzzling colored threads. Because they stained easily with dyes, in 1888 Wilhelm Van Waldeyer would name them "chromosomes," meaning "colored bodies."

Improved staining techniques convinced cytologists that these chromosomes were highly individual and were made up of smaller elements. From 1887–1890, in a series of careful observations of developing eggs of the roundworm *Ascaris*, Theodor Boveri offered proof that the chromosomes were not as supposed a confused, continuous loop, but were individual bodies. Further, he showed that in following the cleavage of the fertilized egg in the young sea urchin embryo it was clear that each new cell had to receive a full set of these threads in order to develop properly.

An extraordinary synthesis had begun to develop. From several decades of painstaking cytological and embryological studies had emerged a picture of microscopic, discrete units within the nucleus of each cell. In cell division these units, the chromosomes, divided longitudinally so that the resulting cells received the same number of chromosomes as the original cell. In fertilization, groups of these chromosomes recombined as the egg and sperm nuclei fused. In 1892 August Weismann could say that "the essence of heredity is the transmission of a nuclear substance of a specific molecular structure," and further that the "sperm and egg cells contain a substance that by the physical and chemical properties of its molecular nature is able to become a new individual of the same species."

But what sounds like a remarkably accurate description of the genes was not that at all. The "unit of heredity" still had not been reduced to anything so specific. Darwinian "gemmules," his imagined invisible particles flowing from all parts of the body to the reproductive organs, had set the tone for a progression of similar inaccurate concepts for many years. These units were thought to serve both as vehicles of transmission as well as directors of development and were assumed to be self-reproducing and to circulate throughout the organism. Herbert Spencer preferred "physiological units," or Naegeli the "ideoplasm." None of these imaginary units were derived from experimental evidence.

It remained for August Weismann, who later would be presented with the Royal Society's Darwin Medal in 1908 as the "one who had done more than any other man to focus attention on the mechanism of inheritance," to break away from these awkward notions and propose that a "germ plasm" made up of the chromosomes was the substance of heredity and that this germ plasm was transmitted from generation to generation. The body, or "soma," he saw as the temporary custodian of their continuous line of germ cells. The determinants of heredity in the chromosomes Weismann described as groups of "ids." These in turn were arranged to consolidate the "idant," or chromosome. While his terminology has long since disappeared, the conviction led Weismann to reject the Lamarckian theory of the inheritance of acquired characteristics which Darwin so begrudgingly had to accept and to center attention on the continuity of chromosomes from parent to offspring and their role in inheritance independent of the rest of the body.

The distinguished Weismann's championing of his concept finally turned scientists in the direction which would eventually lead to the gene. Samuel Butler, the late-nineteenth-century English novelist and essayist, whose hazy notion that inheritance was caused by "unconscious memories" of previous adaptations stirred up little interest among scientists, now turned toward more objective analysis. He was nevertheless strikingly accurate in a remark that he no doubt intended as mere satire: "It has, I believe, been often remarked that a hen is only an egg's way of making another egg."

Butler unwittingly had stated what would not be understood in his lifetime but would become for us part and parcel of our understanding of the function of genes. Stated in modern terms he might have said that the fertilized egg contains a nucleus which is the product of the fusion of the male and female gamete nuclei. Within that nucleus are chromosomes which are made of a long strand of DNA. Some of this DNA acts as genes which contain a code that will direct the egg to divide and eventually form an entire organism, as in the case of the hen. The hen is a highly organized mass of cells, each of which contains the same DNA code which allows the hen to carry out its living functions such as feeding, movement, metabolism, and excretion, all of which operate to support a major function, that of reproduction. In the cell that eventually forms the egg, the nucleus will receive a set of chromosomes, half the number present in the rest of the body's cells. If fertilized, the egg will begin again the ceaseless cycle of development.

But decades would pass before such a scenario would be a commonplace understanding. As the nineteenth century drew to a close, four decades of research centering around the questions posed by Charles Darwin had narrowed the search for the physical vehicle of inheritance to the nucleus. The question remained, as stated by E. B. Wilson in the second (1900) edition of *The Cell in Development and Heredity*, "How do the adult characters lie latent in the germ cell; and how do they become patent as development proceeds?" This is the final question that looms in the background of every investigation of the cell.

The honest answer, as our present century dawned, was "we do not know." But in that very year of 1900 a series of discoveries was to commence that would begin with a remarkable rediscovery. Gregor Mendel would emerge from the shadows. The long overdue recognition of the significance of his brilliant insights would become the cornerstone for the ensuing decades of extraordinary progress which would later lead to the Human Genome Project.

3

FLOWERS, FLIES, MOLDS, AND MICROBES

It might seem to be too facile an approach to divide the history of the search for the gene by merely looking at first the nineteenth- and then the twentieth-century developments. As it turns out, the transition between the last century and the present was marked by a rapid and revolutionary change in the understanding of heredity from that which, despite the remarkable achievements of many scientists, remained a nebulous and controversial series of hypotheses.

The search had narrowed to the nucleus and perhaps to its chromosomes, made up of an acidic substance. These chromosomes had been shown to be passed on to each succeeding generation of cells. How these barely visible objects could actually control the appearance of the organism or even the life of the cell or tissues was baffling. Although the beginning of the study of cells and the attempts at understanding the transmission of characteristics from generation to generation had preceded Darwin, his figure stood like a giant over the nineteenth century. His monumental synthesis of evolutionary theory had stimulated and directed the efforts of a whole generation of scientists toward solving the critical questions that this theory had raised.

As the twentieth century began, a remarkable coincidence soon occurred. Three men, working independently, almost simultaneously rediscovered the work of Gregor Mendel. All of them were also botanists, who themselves had set out to answer the same question that had piqued Mendel's curiosity. Was it possible that there might be a predictable, quantifiable pattern to the inheritance of plant characteristics? In so doing, they came to realize that Mendel had found such a pattern and that this vital information had gone unnoticed for almost 40 years.

One was Hugo De Vries, a botanist from the Netherlands, who during a visit to England during 1877 had been deeply impressed by his conversations with Darwin. He thereafter gradually moved from studies of plant function toward investigation of variation and heredity. De Vries shared the concern of many others that Darwin's ideas of gradual, small changes might not be enough to supply natural selection with enough variation to enable its selective processes eventually to produce major changes in organisms. They also reasoned that, though different and varied offspring certainly could be made by selective breeding experiments, the resulting changes were always only within certain limits and never generated new species.

Also, though Darwin's concept of pangenesis—whereby gemmules acted as particulate units of heredity—appealed to De Vries, he denied that these "pangenes" as he called them could be altered by the environment, thus avoiding the Lamarckian position of Darwin. Instead, he felt that "new kinds of pangenes form" to give variability. In his search for such varied pangenes, he sought for clues in the organisms he knew best, the flowering plants. He wanted to find a clear instance in which he could actually see the development of a new species. In 1866 he found such an example, or so he thought, in a population of the beautiful evening primrose growing abundantly near his home in Amsterdam. The bloom-filled field had spread from displays growing in a cultivated garden in a nearby park. He gathered some, identifying it as *Oenothera lamarckiana*, a species named, ironically, after Jean Baptiste de Lamarck. Over a span of 20 years he raised over 50,000 plants from his original stock. Occasionally he recognized plants that were strikingly different from their parents. New traits in the flowers appeared suddenly, with no clue in their parentage as to where these traits could have arisen from. Significantly these strange plants bred true, that is, these new characteristics persisted when the plants were bred among themselves. Some of these new plants could be crossed with their parents but others could not, leading him to the conviction that they were new species.

A sudden, unpredictable change had occurred. De Vries called these changes mutations and proclaimed that these changes were due to changes in the pangenes. Applied to nature, these changes would be examples of changes in any other organism sufficient to allow natural selection to operate in the spread of this new species.

Unknown to De Vries, he had actually hit upon a principal source of biological variability for which he invented the term "mutation," a term we use to this day. We now know that mutations are molecular changes in genes which can sometimes lead to new characteristics and thus evolution. However, scientists found out many years later that the primrose phenomena were not real mutations at all but new varieties that arose because of a complicated set of events that sometimes occurs in plants; such events include doubling of the chromosome number in the cells, which may produce a "giant," or the loss of half of the chromosomes, which may result in a "dwarf."

Regardless of the mistaken interpretations, in De Vries's breeding work with primroses and many other plant species he was led to some of the same conclusions that Mendel had reached. He realized that inheritance was due to specific units which were passed from parent to offspring in a pattern which could be followed. He pictured the chromatin thread (later to be known as the chromosome) as a place where pangenes were united into groups of various sizes. Further, he saw the splitting of these threads, already established in nineteenth-century cytology as the occasion for the segregation of the pangenes into separate gametes. Each gamete would get a set of pangenes. If the pangenes were in large numbers, they were active and if in smaller numbers, latent. He was wrong about the quantitative effects of his pangenes and never hit upon Mendel's notion of dominant and recessive factors.

Sensing the importance of his work, in 1900 De Vries prepared a lengthy manuscript detailing his findings and conjectures and submitted it to both the French Academy of Sciences and the German Botanical Society. The French paper came out first. One of its readers was a young German, Karl Correns, who read it with what one can suppose was amazement and consternation. Correns had been a student of Karl von Naegeli, to whom Mendel had sent copies of his paper years before. Whether or not Naegeli had mentioned Mendel's notes was never known, but according to Correns's accounts, by October 1899 he had come to recognize, by his own experiments on the inheritance of pea color, the same predictable ratios seen by Mendel. A few weeks after his discovery, which had come to him, as he wrote, "like a flash" as he lay in bed, he had come to read Mendel's paper. He then realized that the "revelation" he had just received had been worked out in masterful fashion 33 years earlier.

Shortly thereafter he read De Vries's accounts and hastily wrote to him, informing him indignantly that De Vries had not referred to the true discoverer of the laws of inheritance, Gregor Mendel, whose paper he certainly must have read. De Vries had in fact read it and was forced to quickly fasten an addendum to his German paper which appeared a few weeks later, indicating that he had "first learned of its existence after I had completed the majority of my experiments and had deduced from them the statements communicated in the text."

Correns, who had earlier decided to forgo releasing his results until they had added more to Mendel's findings, now felt obliged to do so. In his paper, unlike De Vries, he ungrudgingly gave Mendel full credit for his pioneering accomplishments. Years later, in tribute to Mendel, Correns published the series of Mendel's letters which had been sent to Naegeli.

For someone who was unknown for so long, Mendel was suddenly receiving an abundance of recognition. Yet another botanist, Erik von Tshermak-Seysenegg, in the course of experiments to extend Darwin's observations on the effects of self- and cross-fertilization, chose peas because they could be grown quickly in the greenhouse. He discovered the 3:1 ratio and with it the concept of dominance in 1899. While working on his results he came across Mendel's paper. His own publication, as a dissertation, confirmed Mendel's results for single pairs of characters. Coming across the two papers of Correns and De Vries, he then published an abstract of his dissertation in May of 1900. In that same year he arranged to have Mendel's original works published in German.

In that same month in 1900 a Cambridge University biologist had boarded the train for London, where he was to deliver an address to the Royal Horticultural Society on "Problems of Heredity as a Subject for Biological Investigation." He had brought along De Vries's paper for reading material. As the train rumbled along, he read De Vries's accounts of Mendel's laws. From that day, William Bateson devoted his considerable enthusiasm and literary gifts to what he came to call "Mendelism." He immediately had Mendel's paper translated and had it printed with footnotes in the *Journal of the Royal Horticultural Society*. This finally brought Mendel to the attention of the English-speaking world. In Bateson's own words, "His [Mendel's] experiments are worthy to rank with those which laid the foundations of the Atomic laws of Chemistry." His principles were "lying at the very root of all conceptions not merely of the physiology of reproduction and heredity but even of the essential nature of living organisms."

Bateson and several co-workers were soon the first to demonstrate Mendelian principles in animals, for example, poultry. In 1902, Lucien Cuenot showed that certain color "differences" in mice also confirmed Mendel's rules.

Bateson suggested terminology which his contemporaries quickly adopted and which are still in use today. Mendel's pairs of factors, which were actually genes, were to be called "allelomorphs," later shortened to "alleles." The cell formed by union of two gametes, one containing a dominant factor for a particular trait and the other a recessive was called a "heterozygote." If the gametes were similar, that is both having dominant or recessive factors for that trait, it would form a "homozygote." In Bateson's inaugural address to the Third Conference on Hybridization and Plant Breeding on July 31, 1906, he said, "I suggest for the consideration of the Congress the term 'genetics,' which sufficiently indicates that our labours are devoted to the elucidation of the phenomena of heredity and variation . . ."

An extraordinary burst of experimental activity had commenced that by 1920 had solved the fundamental problems of the transmission mechanism of heredity. The first decade of the century had come to be known as the Age of Mendelism, sparked by the fervor of Bateson's attention centered on Mendel's principles. At the very same time cytological studies, carried on since Mendel's time, had amassed sufficient information to quickly allow a key synthesis. August Weismann and others had readily established that during the formation of gametes (the process of meiosis) all of the chromosomes in the cells producing the gametes separate into equal numbers. Each gamete (sperm or egg) therefore received half of the original number of chromosomes ordinarily found in the cells of those organisms. Two investigators, Theodor Boveri in Germany and Walter Sutton in Columbia University in New York, first called attention to this movement of chromosomes in meiosis and thus the separation of Mendelian factors associated with those chromosomes.

Sutton, while still a young graduate student, had been busy studying the chromosomes in the testes of grasshoppers, collected from his father's wheat fields in Kansas. The chromosomes were large and variously shaped and their fate could be followed by squashing and staining these dividing cells. He concluded in December 1902 in the *Biological Bulletin* that chromosomes reside in cells as look-alike pairs. One member of each pair was "paternal" having been originally contributed by the male parent and the other "maternal," derived from the female parent. At meiosis, these pairs separated and each gamete received only one member, either paternal or maternal, of those original pairs. He pointed out that this "may constitute the physical basis of Mendelian heredity." Moreover, in 1903 he expanded on his original observations and added that in meiosis each member of these chromosome pairs presses very close to its partner. They then separate from each other and the maternal and paternal chromosomes move into the gametes randomly.

Thus the gametes always have the same number of chromosomes, but of those, the number of chromosomes of maternal or paternal origin is variable. Boveri, working with sea urchins, had reached the same conclusion. Historians argue over who should receive precedence in recognition and we read variously of the "Sutton–Boveri" or the "Boveri–Sutton" theory but clearly both had finally found a home for the gene.

Whatever it was, the gene, which somehow influenced whatever characters one could see and perhaps invisible ones as well, must reside in the chromosomes, those threads of nuclein and protein. Boveri wrote of these threads in 1903: "We eventually want to know what in fact these chromatin elements which bear such remarkable destinies possess in respect of physiological signficance."

There now appeared to be a quite logical connection between chromosomes and Mendel's hereditary factors. However, many would not agree that the relationship was more than coincidental without further proof. Among the dissenters was William Bateson, Mendel's proselyte, and another man as well, who would soon become one of the leading geneticists of this century.

Thomas Hunt Morgan had begun his career as an embryologist, devising experiments to test theories of how the developing egg produces a complex organism with differentiated structure, a problem we might add that still perplexes us even today. Morgan had joined the faculty of Bryn Mawr as a young professor in 1891, the same year that Jacques Loeb arrived there from Germany. Loeb's strong mechanist influence drew Morgan toward an emphasis of the chemical and physical processes expressing themselves as life. Morgan came to Columbia in 1902. He had long been uncomfortable with the fact that the relationship between factors and chromosomes was basically inferential and demanded experimental proof. He was also interested in replacing Darwin's hazy notion of variation with the more recent concept, also undefined, of mutation, as proposed by De Vries, whose lab he had visited in 1903.

Edmond B. Wilson, his new colleague, had created a unique course, which was immediately oversubscribed. It dealt with the emerging synthesis of heredity, chromosomes, variation, and evolution. The best and the brightest enthusiasts in this course went on to further study, where they were welcomed by Morgan, a superb teacher and motivator. They formed an incredibly productive partnership, which established, through a series of brilliant experiments carried out by the students, the very theories which Morgan had earlier found unsatisfactory.

Between 1910 and 1925, a small, crowded laboratory at Columbia and during the summer months a similar room at Woods Hole were the homes for several generations of students lucky enough to be admitted to this cluttered inner sanctum. The students willingly shared their limited space with hundreds and eventually thousands of glass milk bottles, which reeked with the smell of rotting bananas, food for *Drosophila*, otherwise known as the common fruit fly.

This diminutive creature now ranks among the most intensively studied of all living organisms, but in 1910 it was a comparative newcomer to the world of science. An entymologist friend, Frank Lutz, suggested that the fly might prove useful as an experimental tool. After all, *Drosophila*, given a little food and warmth, would oblige by producing a new generation every two weeks. Only eight hours after emergence the tiny new flies would begin to mate. A little ether to anesthetize the flies, a bit of dexterity, and a magnifying lens could serve to separate males from unmated females. Controlled matings of flies with specific characteristics could then be carried out. Perhaps some of De Vries's mutations might show up in some easily detectable characteristic of the fly, such as wing shape or eye color. Such mutations might then somehow be linked to the four chromosomes known to be in each fly cell.

Months of patient breeding and rearing of flies proved "fruitless." And then one day in 1910, a single and singular male fly appeared in a culture bottle. Unlike the thousands of its predecessors, who had red eyes (really quite beautiful when seen through a microscope), its eyes were white. Morgan immediately mated the prized male with a normal red-eyed female, following the approach that Mendel had established. The white-eyed male, a bit sluggish before the mating, quietly expired. But he had done all that was necessary. All of the 1237 flies that resulted had red eyes. Flies from this first generation were crossed among themselves and as hoped, a 3:1 ratio of red eyes to white constituted the second generation. It appeared that red was dominant over the recessive white. Something was strange, however, about these results. Unpredictable by Mendel's theory, all of the white-eyed flies were males!

Morgan quickly turned to the current information on *Drosophila* chromosomes. Betty Stevens, a student of Morgan's when he was at Bryn Mawr, had searched painstakingly through various tissues of *Drosophila* in a search for chromosomes. She discovered that if she dissected out the two large salivary glands from the late larval stage, a squashed and stained preparation showed eight remarkably large chromosomes, much larger than found in any of the other cells. Importantly, in males, one of the pairs did not match. One chromosome was straight and the other had a distinct bend or hook. The female always had two of the straight, labeled X chromosomes and the male had one X and one bent, the Y.

Could this odd Y chromosome determine the sex of the male fly? And if it did, was a factor inducing eye color lacking on this smaller chromosome, so that males would always exhibit the expression of whatever eye color factor might be on the X chromosome? If so, then the eggs of XX females, which could only produce X-containing gametes, would have to be fertilized by a Y chromosome in order to produce a male. If the X chromosome had on it a dominant factor governing red eyes, the male would be red-eyed. Only if the recessive white factor were on the X chromosome would the fly appear as a white-eyed male. In an XX female combination the expression of a recessive white-eyed factor on one X chromosome would usually be masked by the much more common, dominant red-eyed factor on the other X. Only in rare instances would the sperm and egg both carry an X chromosome bearing a recessive eye gene. Could a recessive gene on each of the two X chromosomes result in a white-eyed female? Further breeding experiments proved that this was exactly what appeared to be happening. It was a stunning discovery. Sutton and Boveri had been correct. Chromosomes do carry the heredity factors and some of those factors determine sexuality.

Serendipity turned into the order of the day as new and varied mutations sprung up in the fly cultures. Morgan welcomed two Columbia University students into his laboratory, Alfred E. Sturtevant and Calvin B. Bridges. Soon they had spotted other "sex-linked" recessive characters such as abnormally small wings or yellow body color. Bridges was particular adept at cataloging mutants and soon scores of bottles housed useful mutants, ranging from flies with branched bristles, irregular wing veins, and various striped markings. As their breeding crosses multiplied it quickly became apparent that most of these traits were not associated with the X chromosome; in fact they had nothing at all to do with the sex of the fly. It became evident that a mere eight chromosomes would certainly have to carry many more than one factor each to account for such a diversity of characteristics. It also made sense in theory and was obvious in practice that the factors which resided on the same chromosome would be inherited together.

Gradually, particularly through the labors of another student, Herman J. Muller, four distinct groups of mutants emerged. One of these groups numbered only a few compared to the other three and appeared to correspond to the smallest of the four pairs of chromosomes. The evidence was overwhelming. Factors must be located on specific chromo-

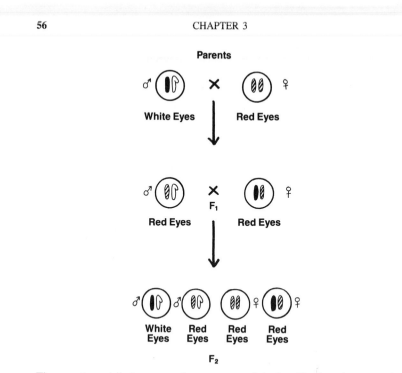

The parents contribute one sex chromosome each to the offspring. A gene on the solid chromosome results in white eyes—if the bent chromosome is present, as in the male. A female would need two of the solid chromosomes in order to have white eyes.

somes. Each factor was inherited only if the sperm or egg happened to contain that member of the chromosome pair where that factor was located. Since the chromosomes were long threads, were those factors strung on the filaments like the pearls on a string? No one knew, nor did there appear to be any available way to find out, for the factors, whatever they were, were invisible.

Meanwhile these Mendelian factors finally received a permanent, more descriptive name. In 1909 Wilhelm Johannsen, a Danish plant physiologist, offered a convenient terminology for the new discipline of genetics, named earlier by Bateson. He settled on the last syllable of pangene, which De Vries had taken from Darwin's theory of pangenesis. Factors would be called "genes," the set of genes governing a characteristic of an individual, for example, its color, would be its "genotype" for that characteristic. The trait itself would be called a "phenotype." The elusive factors had a name, a gene, and genes had a home on the chromosome. But what was a gene?

Alfred Sturtevant was puzzled. The four neat stacks of mutants assigned to the four chromosome pairs showed some annoying inconsistencies. Genes which had been shown to be linked together on the same chromosome occasionally seemed to show up in the wrong place and appeared to be now located on a different chromosome. He knew that only a few years earlier, in 1909, a paper by the Belgian cytologist F. A. Jannsens had included a description of amphibian chromosome preparations which, during gamete formation (meiosis), showed distinct overlapping, or crossed chromosomes, which he had labeled chiasmata.

Jannsens interpreted this phenomena as an actual fusion of two chromosomes followed by breakage and reunion leading to an exchange of corresponding chromosome regions. This would allow the possibility of genes normally on one chromosome to end up on another. This conclusion was entirely theoretical but Sturtevant and Morgan seized upon it as a possible explanation of the unsettling exceptions to their neat scheme of linked genes. If this actually occurred, common sense told them that genes farther apart on the chromosomes would certainly have a greater chance than genes located close together of being exchanged as the chromosomes crossed over, broke, and recombined.

Sturtevant immediately devised experiments with this theory in mind and by 1913 had shown that six genes, all located on the X chromosome, did indeed appear to occasionally be interchanged during meiosis. In so doing he had produced the first chromosome map. The six genes could be arranged on the X chromosome on the basis of their crossing-over frequencies in a linear order.

It would be 15 years before John Stern would actually prove directly in 1931 that physical interchange could be followed in microscopic preparations, but a major milestone had been reached. Morgan and his co-workers had firmly established that genes were arranged on the chromosomes in a linear order. The phenomenon of crossing-over during gamete formation could lead to even greater variability in the offspring beyond that afforded by the recombination of the sperm and egg.

In other words, meiosis, in which chromosomes of paternal and maternal origin were parceled out at random into the gametes was not the only source of variation in the characteristics of offspring. Crossing-over made many other combinations of genetic messages to add to those variations. Not only were Mendel's conjectures supported more fully than ever, but to the search for the source of variation and evolution was added a new arrival, crossing-over.

Soon maps of other *Drosophila* chromosomes were made, based on the principle that map distance was related to the distance between the genes. Ever since Sturtevant developed his simple but important map, linkage maps have been essential tools for many genetic analyses. The first major genetic linkage map marking the relative position of 403 genes in humans was published in 1987. One ambitious goal of the HGP is the completion, in 1995, of a much more highly detailed human genetic map.

Still, there is not a single organism whose chromosomes have been completely mapped. And what of *Drosophila*? Almost eight decades have passed since Alfred Sturtevant sketched out his string of six lone genes along the length of an X chromosome. The *Drosophila* genome map has not as yet been completed. The fruit fly waits humbly in line

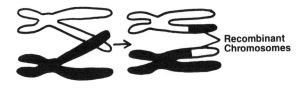

Crossing–over

Here, each chromosome has made a replicate and the two are still attached, so they appear as an X shape. As the cell divides to make gametes, pieces of the chromosomes overlap and literally exchange parts. Each of these four chromosomes will end up in a separate gamete.

with a few other candidates, a bacterium, a weed, and a worm, seeking to become the model organism for large-scale genome mapping in cooperation with the Human Genome Project.

In 1915 the classic book, *The Mechanism of Mendelian Heredity*, co-authored by Morgan, Sturtevant, Bridges, and Muller, made the cluttered fly room the world center of genetic research. It was a triumph for mechanistic methodology. Morgan would receive the Nobel prize in 1933 for developing the chromosome theory of heredity. In one sense, the search for the gene had ended in that it had finally passed beyond the realm of theory and had been experimentally demonstrated to be a physical entity on the chromosome. In a real sense, however, the search had only begun, because the essential mystery remained. What was a gene? What could its presence possibly have to do with the corresponding presence of a character, such as red eyes in a fly or the color and shape of peas in a pod? Mendelism had replaced the vague notions of homunculus, gemmules, or ids but no more was known about specifically how or why these genes worked.

This seemingly intractable puzzle was solved only as the nature of genes on chromosomes began to be seen in dynamic rather than static terms. A major impetus for such a change in perspective was provided by Herman Muller when he began to take a critical look at the underlying causes for all those occasional unpredictable but wonderfully convenient phenotype changes in *Drosophila* which had led the fly room group to their dramatic findings. True, they were assumed to be caused by mutations now considered a change in a gene but it could only be an act of the imagination to describe any modifications in a structure of which nothing was known in the first place. In 1921, after Muller had left Columbia and was working independently, he stated, "Beneath the imposing structure called Heredity there has been a dingy basement called Mutations." Muller, a careful and precise researcher, set out to answer a specific question: Could mutations be deliberately induced and accurately and quantitatively identified?

De Vries, as far back as 1904, had suggested in a lecture at the Station for Experimental Evolution at Cold Spring Harbor that the "rays of Roentgen" which were able to penetrate into the interior of living tissue might be used in an attempt to alter the hereditary particles of mature cells. Muller was not the first to try to induce hereditary changes in cells but the few others who attempted this had produced no clear results. Muller possessed a crucial advantage, his long experience with an experimental system, the fruit fly.

The rays of Roentgen were X rays which were first produced in 1895. Madame Curie and her husband Pierre had also discovered another kind of short-wave high-energy radiation that emanated from radioactive elements such as radium. These rays could easily penetrate all but the densest material such as lead. All the awesome destructive force of radiation was not yet fully appreciated, but it seemed to Muller a likely candidate for a powerful enough tool, for the radiation penetrated deep into cells and perhaps could affect genes.

He began by determining the low measurable mutation rates in the X chromosomes induced by temperature changes. It was already known that these mutations were lethal, that is, they would kill the male flies. Such mutations occurred at the rate of 2 to 5 per 10,000 X chromosomes tested. Exposure to X rays not only dramatically increased the rate of mutations over that occurring because of temperature changes, but significantly the mutation frequently was proportional to the intensity of the radiation applied. Not only that, a cornucopia of mutations were induced by X rays. The genes had been changed by the simple expedient of bombarding them with short-wave energy. This was quite quickly confirmed in other laboratories with both animals and plants and a new discipline was born, that of "radiation genetics."

The gene, whose molecular structure was still unknown, was most evidently real. One could now hit it with a whole spectrum of projectiles and these collisions could produce a change in the gene to make it act differently. Moreover, it appeared that genes differed in size, since larger genes were hit more often and were changed more frequently than presumably smaller genes. Mutations would now be the means, as Muller put it in 1923, for an "alteration of the gene." The mutant gene, so patiently gathered one by one over the years by Morgan and his students, could now be induced by the hundreds. They would become an essential basic tool of modern gene research. Yet another Nobel prize in genetic research went to Muller in 1946.

Shortly after the rediscovery of Mendel, several papers appeared in medical journals, authored by Archibald E. Garrod, a professor of medicine at Oxford. He claimed to have had discovered a demonstrable example of inherited Mendelian recessive factors while tracing a rare disease through several generations of human families. One of these was the condition of alkaptonuria, an otherwise harmless but bizarre condition in which individuals' urine turned black on exposure to air. Such a phenomenon hardly escaped notice and allowed Dr. Garrod to trace its pedigree back through several generations. In so doing, he found that the incidence was highest in first-cousin marriages. He reasoned, with the help of his friend and colleague William Bateson, that this was quite consistent with the increased possibility of two recessive factors being recombined in the offspring of closely related individuals. The actual defect of alkaptonuria was shown to be traceable to a metabolic problem. It looked as though it resulted from the lack of a particular enzyme, which allowed homogentisic acid, normally broken down by the cells, to build up and spill over into the urine.

By the early twentieth century, a great deal of information had been amassed by chemists about the major building blocks of cells. Büchner, in 1897, showed that even solutions extracted from cells could convert sugar to alcohol. It had been well established that chemical processes of cells were controlled by enzymes and that these enzymes, though diverse, were always proteins. Chemical information ultimately would combine with microscopic, cytological, and functional data to draw a clear picture of the true nature of the gene.

Garrod was clearly too far ahead of his time. In 1908 his series of lectures "Inborn Errors of Metabolism" created little stir. His insights into the role of genes in living systems had been extraordinarily accurate. The concept of genes, at that time still called factors, as inherited particles whose presence in a dominant form could cause enzyme production and whose presence in the double recessive condition prevented an enzyme from being produced is our modern explanation of alkaptonuria. Despite Bateson's support, there were few takers.

L.T. Troland, a physicist remarking upon the state of biology in 1917, stated in an essay in *American Naturalist*: "Men eminent in biology seem to quake before the complexity and delicacy of life processes.

Despite the increasing amount of information gathered by scientists, there is a rejuvenation of mysticism and Aristotelian teleology." Masses of new data were being compiled, particularly about the chemistry of living cells. With the inability of scientists to synthesize this information into a coherent picture, vitalism seemed to some to take on renewed credibility. But eventually the mechanistic approach would prevail, for as Harvard's George Wald has said, "No great idea is ever lost. Like Anteus it is overthrown only to rise again with renewed vigour."

Thomas Hunt Morgan again entered the picture. He had left Columbia for Cal Tech in 1927 where he and Sturtevant had been invited to form a Division of Biology, a novel integrative attempt to abolish the traditional departmental separations of zoology, botany, and microbiology. George Beadle, a doctoral student working under Sturtevant, became interested in working out the genetic details of eye color in *Drosophila*. In 1920 Sturtevant had hypothesized that this process might be due to a diffusible substance within the tissues during eye formation.

Beadle traveled to Paris to work with Boris Euphressi and his new techniques for transplanting potential eye tissue of *Drosophila* larval stages into new larval hosts. Their delicate work suggested the principle that a biochemical substance within the host larva could influence the eye color of the transplanted larval tissue. Analysis of their findings suggested that a series of discrete biochemical steps led up to eye pigment formation. A mutant fly gene resulted in the inability of the tissues to make a particular enzyme during a specific step in that chain. They admitted that such a conclusion was purely a gratuitous assumption.

Understandably elated but equally frustrated by the technical difficulties of isolating from the mass of fly larval tissue specific enzymes controlled by a hypothetical gene, Beadle returned to California where he joined Edward L. Tatum, another chemist. They knew a simpler organism had to be found. *Drosophila* had taken over almost every genetic lab in the world but even the tiny fly was an enormously complicated biochemical system. In a purely pragmatic sense, they needed a living laboratory simple enough to convincingly confirm their tentative hypothesis of one gene producing one enzyme whose function expressed itself as a visible characteristic.

The always-helpful Morgan had brought a culture of the red mold

Neurospora with him to California. It had been given to him by Bernard O. Dodge, who had worked out its life cycle with the suggestion that it might prove to be a useful tool in genetic studies. Beadle had recalled a lecture by Dodge which he had attended and considered that certain characteristics of this now-available organism might lend itself to the question at hand. This fateful decision, based on these chance circumstances, led Beadle and Tatum to win a Nobel prize in 1958. Within a few years, *Drosophila*, although still widely used, would no longer be the geneticists' organism of choice.

Neurospora had a number of useful features. Instead of reproducing in the two weeks that it took *Drosophila*, the fungus could produce a new generation of thousands of individuals in a few hours. When seen through the microscope, such molds appear to be abundantly branched fine filaments of cells arranged end to end in a single row. These filaments when not reproducing by sexual means can propagate themselves asexually by simply subdividing into many thousands of small, spherical cells called "spores." Each spore contains only half of the full set of chromosomes that are present after the fungus fuses in sexual reproduction. In other words, it contains one of each of the original pairs of chromosomes just as a gamete does. This means that if a recessive gene is present it can express itself because there is no chance that a dominant gene somewhere on the other member of the chromosome pair would overcome it.

The fungus grows easily in test tubes or plates with artificial food of known composition in the lab. *Neurospora* needs only a little nitrate, phosphate, sulphate, glucose, and a single vitamin, biotin. With these building blocks the fungus can synthesize all of the carbohydrates, fats, proteins, and vitamins that it needs.

Fungi in general have evolved over their billions of years of existence to be extraordinarily self-sufficient. That implied, Beadle and Tatum reasoned, that its genes could easily bring into being all the enzymes necessary for its metabolism. In a definitive experiment, spores were first irradiated with X rays and then individual spores were placed into separate tubes of a rich medium. The spores grew into a mass of filaments, a "mycelium." When transferred to a very simple medium, the bits of mycelium, each the descendants of a simple spore, grew as well as before, that is, all but culture number 299 out of the 1000 cultures initiated. It was unable to grow unless the mycelium was placed on a medium containing pyridoxine (vitamin B6). If the hypothesis was correct, the irradiation had mutated a gene and it could no longer cause the production of an enzyme necessary to help synthesize pyridoxine. Thus it would then have to be supplied from an external source. Further experiments uncovered X-ray-induced mutants which, while they could synthesize pyridoxine, were not able to synthesize one or more other metabolic substances.

These "deficiency mutations," as they were called, appeared to have a genetic basis. If this were so, then the altered gene should pass on to another generation. The mycelium from a mutated strain of mold was crossed with another normal strain. In primitive organisms there are no gametes such as sperm and egg. Cells of the filaments themselves fuse and form a mycelium which undergoes meiosis to produce great masses of spores. The descendants of these spores showed a clear Mendelian segregation. Half of the spores could grow like the normal parent strain and the other half needed pyridoxine in the medium.

Beadle and Tatum had proved that a mutation could result in a nutritional deficiency and this loss of an ability to perform a biochemical reaction was due to a heritable gene alteration. Their stunning synthesis is known in the lore of biology as the "one gene, one enzyme hypothesis." One gene defect prevented one enzyme from being made. It was an enormous achievement which brought about the union of genetics, microbiology, biochemistry, and developmental biology—a powerfully productive coalition. It established the attitude toward the gene as something that was able to direct the synthesis of an enzyme (a protein) and thus forged the link between the still enigmatic hereditary particle and the maze of biochemical reactions which constitute life itself. In his Nobel lecture, Beadle pointed out that although he and his colleagues had not known of Garrod's work during the time of their experiments, "we had rediscovered what Garrod had seen so clearly so many years before."

The chromosomes were known to be a mixture of nucleic acid and protein. The genes were part of that worrisome complex chemical mix. The genes were somehow making enzymes which were active in the cytoplasm, that region between the nucleus and the cell membrane.

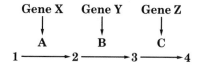

Each of these three chemical reactions (1–2, 2–3, 3–4) needs a different enzyme (A, B, or C). Each enzyme is made according to directions from a different gene.

Between 1926 and 1930 James Sumner of Cornell University and John Northrop of the Rockefeller Institute had proven conclusively that all enzymes were proteins. The triumphs of mechanism always seemed to raise more questions than they answered. Biological reductionism had arrived at the gene as chemical. Only its molecular details could reveal precisely how it functioned. Since proteins were so complex and all nucleic acid was assumed to be alike regardless of whatever oganism it was extracted from, the nuclear protein seemed to be the best candidate for the office of gene. The incredible variety of enzymes needed by cells could hardly be supplied by a molecule of homogeneous composition nor could the different enzyme requirements of all the earth's species be met by such a molecule. How could a gene which was a protein make yet another completely different protein?

A major part of the puzzle was soon solved. In 1913, a young physician, Oswald Avery, had been recruited by the Rockefeller Institute in New York City to pursue his research there on respiratory diseases. The Institute was founded in 1901 when John D. Rockefeller, Sr., after losing a grandchild from scarlet fever, established the research complex to study causes of infectious disease. Lewis Thomas describes Avery as a "small, vanishingly thin man with a constantly startled expression and a very large and agile brain." After graduating from medical school he soon gave up the practice of clinical medicine, which at that time, despite the invention of anesthesia and a growing respect for aseptic technique, had almost nothing to offer in the way of cures, particularly in the case of infections, such as tuberculosis, pneumonia, smallpox, tetanus, or diphtheria.

He turned to research on pneumonia, a perennial killer, particularly of both the very young and very old. Certain forms of pneumonia were known to be caused by the pneumococcus bacterium, and in his search through the literature on the subject he was beguiled by some experiments with the very same organism in 1928 by Frederick Griffith, a British Public Health Service scientist. Griffith knew that this bacterium was found in two forms, the usual smooth "S" form, whose cells formed sticky carbohydrate capsules around themselves, and a rare rough "R" form, whose cells lacked this covering. Somehow the capsules blocked the body's defenses against the encroachment of the bacteria, for when he injected them (the "S" cells) into mice, they induced a fatal pneumonia. Injections of the "R" form were harmless, however.

Intrigued, Griffith next injected mice with the "S" infective forms after first killing the bacteria with heat. As he expected, the mice were not harmed. He then injected more of these heat-killed "S" cells along with a dose of live "R"-type noninfective bacteria. All of the mice died and upon autopsy were found to be filled with live "S" bacteria! Astonished, Griffith repeated his experiments many times, always with identical results. Somehow a substance in the dead cells must have entered the live "R" cells, thus transforming them into cells capable of making the protective carbohydrate capsule. In this protected state they could cause a lethal pneumonia.

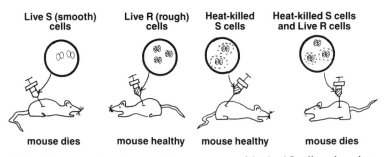

The live R cells are "transformed" by the presence of the dead S cells and are then able to cause pneumonia.

He was met with almost universal skepticism. His cause was not helped by the fact that he was even more self-effacing than Avery. He was so shy that he could not even manage to read his papers in front of audiences. Given this, he was hardly one to champion his cause, à la Bateson or Morgan. However, the objections were not without foundation. After all, Griffith was claiming that something had been released from dead bacteria which caused a change in live bacteria which was passed on to all of their descendants.

Avery took Griffith at his word and set out to determine what the transforming principle might be. He would report during the ensuing years that "disappointment was my daily bread." Working first with Colin MacLeod and then with MacLyn McCarty, he showed that crude extracts of the dead cells brought about the transformation, but the extract was a complex mixture of carbohydrates, lipids, proteins, nucleic acids, and other constituents. Patiently they eliminated first one ingredient and then another. In 1944 they had the answer. When the transforming principle was purified as far as their methods allowed, it consisted predominantly of DNA, referred to by Avery as "thymus nucleic acid." All but trace amounts of protein, 0.02%, could be removed without lowering the transformation efficiency.

In 1945, the now-renowned H.J. Muller championed the humble Avery's cause. He said that, "In my opinion, the most probable interpretation becomes the actual entrance of the foreign genetic material. Parts of chromosomes have penetrated the capsule-less bacteria and taken root there, perhaps having undergone a kind of crossing-over with the chromosomes of the hosts." The inference was, of course, that the genes were actually transferred from the dead "S" cells to the live "R" cells, changing them into "S" cells. Those genes were DNA and the DNA could mingle and combine with the genes of the host DNA, conferring a new trait, that of capsule making. The scientific community was impressed but not entirely convinced. Chemical theory still pointed to proteins as genes. After all, were bacterial chromosomes really comparable to human or other more highly advanced chromosomes?

As it turned out, Avery was correct. Confirmation of his pioneering work soon followed from a quite unexpected source. What resulted was an entirely new field of life sciences known as molecular biology, the discipline in which most of those who are undertaking the Human Genome Project work. Nonetheless, the Nobel prize eluded the self-effacing Avery. It went instead to a team of men, brilliant in their own right, who later confirmed beyond doubt what the diminutive scientist with the "very large and agile brain" had already discovered. As for Griffith, he never learned of Avery's explanation of his findings. He was dead, killed by bombs falling on London during World War II. He had refused to leave his laboratory during an air raid.

As the search for the gene expanded, the living organisms used as tools in that search grew smaller. Flowering plants had given way to fruit flies, then to fungi, and finally bacteria. No other living creature could match the bacteria in the size of the populations that could be produced in the lab. A single cell under good conditions could divide into two every 20 minutes and overnight more bacteria could be raised in a few flasks than all the fruit flies that had ever lived. The only thing smaller than bacteria that contained DNA were viruses.

Their existence had been known since 1883, when the German botanist A. Mayer searched for the cause of tobacco mosaic disease, which stunted the growth of the plants and gave the leaves a mottled, or mosaic coloration. The disease could be transmitted when the sap from infected leaves was sprayed onto healthy plants. However, the sap contained no bacteria. A decade later the Russian scientist D. Ivanowski passed infected sap through a porcelain filter that could remove all bacteria. This filtered sap was still infective. Whatever the mysterious agent was it could not be cultivated on growth media, although it obviously reproduced in the plant, since it could be passed along through many generations of plants.

The American Wendel M. Stanley finally isolated the infectious particle in 1935. Amazingly, he extracted it from solutions by crystallization. These "filterable viruses" as they were called were not living organisms at all. When the crystals were redissolved their infectious properties were intact. These data could not be ignored but what could one do with them?

Scientists began to reflect on the long-neglected work of the Canadian Felix D'Herelle, who in 1912 had isolated viruses that could infect and destroy bacteria. A turbid suspension of bacterial cells, once exposed to these agents, would turn clear in just a few hours. A few drops of the clear culture transferred to a new bacterial suspension would have the same effect. These invisible killers could be propagated indefinitely. Initial enthusiasm for these as agents to combat infectious disease waned as this proved impractical. The bacteria predators, which he called "bacteriophages" (literally "bacteria eaters" or "phages"), for convenience remained as curiosities.

Then, in 1934, Martin Schlesinger announced that a chemical analysis of bacteriophages revealed that they consisted of nucleic acid and protein. As yet, no one had ever seen a virus. They are far below the limits of resolution of light microscopes, the smallest being 50 times less than that of the typical bacterial cell. The electron microscope, capable of fully revealing their structure, was not invented until 1933 and in 1939 the tobacco mosaic virus was the first virus ever to be seen.

A group of scientists, headed by Max Delbrück, Salvador Luria, and Alfred Hershey began to speculate that perhaps the use of these viruses might finally constitute a system where one could study the activity of DNA versus that of proteins. Their work was centered at Cold Spring Harbor Laboratories, which at that time was divided between the Biological Laboratories and the Carnegie Institute of Genetics. The latter had come to Cold Spring Harbor in 1902 and had already been the site of the development of hybrid corn, which formed the basis of modern agriculture and is considered one of the greatest biological discoveries of this century.

In 1939 Max Delbrück and Emily Ellis had shown that certain bacteriophages actually multiplied inside bacteria cells and that the cells released these progeny when they split open. Thomas Anderson and Salvador Luria obtained the first electron microscope pictures of a bacteriophage in 1942. Delbrück introduced a summer course on phages at Cold Spring Harbor in 1945. Attracted by the presence of a distinguished faculty and the lure of spending a few weeks in the idyllic seaside setting, doubly enhanced by the fervor and camaraderie of the participants, students thronged to Cold Spring Harbor from all over the world each year. This "phage group," as it has come to be called, was the intellectual watershed of molecular biology. Many of its participants went on to accomplishments which would lay the foundations for the work of the molecular study of life as we now practice it. They would also later contribute, personally or through their students, to the birth of the Human Genome Project.

A particular phage came into frequent use because it attached to the bacterium *Escherichia coli*, a common intestinal bacterium. These phages were labeled T2, T4, and T6 or, for convenience, the T-even phages. In the 1940s the electron microscope had been developed to the point where other viruses could now be seen. Unlike light microscopy with which one can directly view objects by peering through a lens system, electron microscopy does not involve looking directly at a specimen. Instead, this massive highly technical system hurls narrow beams of electrons down through a vacuum tube on to the metal-coated specimens. Most electrons pass through but some strike them and are reflected at various angles. These are captured on a screen which projects an image from which one can then generate photographs.

The T phages turned out to have a remarkably complex and unexpected shape. At one end is a hexagonal "head" and on the other a protruding "tail" with fibers extending from the tail. When a suspension of these phages is mixed with a culture of *Escherichia coli*, the phages can be seen to be attached to the wall of the bacterial cells in great numbers. About 20 minutes later, something spectacular happens. The bacteria burst open and about 100 complete new viruses are released while the original infecting viruses are still clinging to the cell exterior. Clearly some influence passes from the phage to the particles to the cell where it causes the formation of living viruses.

When phages are diluted in water, they burst and their contents are liberated. Their hexagonal coat or the tail can be separated by centrifugation and chemical analysis shows that those fragments at the bottom of the centrifuge tubes are proteins. What had been inside of the head is DNA.

In 1952, at Cold Spring Harbor, Alfred Hershey and Martha Chase took advantage of yet another technological breakthrough. DNA was known to contain phosphorus but no sulfur. On the other hand, protein contains some sulfur but no phosphorus. Both phosphorus and sulfur could now be obtained in radioactive form. Hershey and Chase first grew *E. coli* in nutrient solution containing either radioactive phosphate or

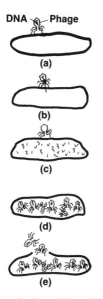

(a) The bacteriophage lands on the bacterial cell, (b) injects DNA, (c,d) new bacteriophages are made, and (e) the cell bursts, releasing the new viruses.

sulfate. Such radioactive forms are known as isotopes, in this case called ^{35}S or ^{32}P for radioactive sulfur and phosphorus. They infected the resulting radioactively labeled bacteria with unlabeled T2 phage. A few generations of viral infections resulted in a suspension of T2 whose DNA or protein was radioactive. These T2 phages were then used to infect a separate suspension of ordinary unlabeled *E. coli* cells.

The next problem was to subject these millions of bacterial cells, upon which were clinging the now-radioactive viruses, to shear forces sufficient to tear the phages away from the cell wall. First, however, they needed sufficient time to pass whatever stimulus they could to the host bacteria. Nothing seemed to work until another new technology of a less than precise nature saved the day. The new technology was provided by the use of a simple kitchen blender. Fred Waring, a popular band leader of the 1950s, had invented the kitchen blender which now bears his name.

The blender, devised for cooks to chop, purée, or otherwise punish food, was tried almost as a last resort. A few minutes of violent agitation in the blender broke the particles loose from the bacterial walls and the two could be separated by centrifugation.

When the bacteria had been infected with the phage containing labeled protein, most of the radioactivity was found in the fraction that contained virus particles. This suggested that the protein did not enter the bacterial cells. The bacteria that had been infected with the phage containing radioactive DNA yielded, after centrifugation, a pellet of bacterial cells showing radioactivity. Moreover, when these bacteria were put back into culture medium they soon burst and released phages containing radioactive phosphorus.

The experiment was definitive, though as usual healthy skepticism produced a rash of questions, repetitions, and refinements of these experiments. Nothing contradicted the evidence that DNA had been injected by the phage into the host bacterial cells while the protein remained outside. The genetic information brought into the bacteria had directed them to manufacture many new bacteriophages. The DNA was in fact an informational macromolecule. The 1969 Nobel prize was shared by Delbrück and Luria.

Science had arrived at the gene and it was DNA. But how could DNA contain enough varied information literally to control the life of an organism? Moreover, how could it replicate and pass itself along cell after cell and retain the message?

Salvadore Luria was convinced that the answer could only come when the exact three-dimensional molecular structure of DNA was known. Not a chemist himself, Luria decided to send one of his students who had just received his Ph.D. to do postdoctoral research in Copenhagen with Herman Kalckar, a chemist who had taken the phage course in 1945. The student he had in mind was definitely bright but his interest in chemistry up to that point had been less than intense. But Luria sent him off, hoping that the Copenhagen lab would yield the synthesis of chemistry and genetics that would finally lead to the understanding of the gene. The student's name was James Watson.

4

DNA: MODELS AND MEANING

Through observation, experimentation, and inspired speculation, what at first were vague and inchoate notions of the gene became increasingly more finely focused. Still, despite accurate conclusions being drawn about the gene—its location in the chromosome and its key role in the life of the cell and in heredity—the molecular architecture and exact function of the gene remained mysteries until halfway through the twentieth century. In our telling of the tale of the penetration of those mysteries we need to introduce some technical details here. These details center around the DNA molecule and its activities within the cell.

In fact, these are the technicalities that one must grasp in order to understand the current interpretation of the human genome. They must be understood to appreciate, beyond simple generalities, how the growing information about the genome can first be interpreted meaningfully and then applied to manipulate genes for scientific and medical purposes. Such an understanding has become a common denominator among biologists. It must be as well for all others who want to have an informed insight into how and why the knowledge derived from this analysis will have such a profound impact on not only human but on all living systems.

With the work of Watson and his colleagues, a golden age of molecular biology would begin. New technologies would be spawned to carry forth the expansion of knowledge about the functions of the gene. The Human Genome Project has become possible only because of this array of developments. Its tools and methodologies are in great measure those initiated in the 1950s through the 1970s. The new era began with what is considered to be the most significant synthesis in the biological sciences since the work of Charles Darwin. We refer to the story of the "double helix."

James Dewey Watson was always bright. He had been one of the original "Quiz Kids" on the wartime radio program and had entered the University of Chicago at the age of 15. Although he could not have known it at the time, the University was then the site of the world's first "atomic pile." As part of the Manhattan Project the top secret "pile" was a gigantic stack of graphite blocks enclosing rods of uranium. The clandestine pile, unknown even to the president of the University, had been assembled under the stands of the unused football stadium.

On December 2, 1942, under the watchful eye of Enrico Fermi, designer of the pile, cadmium control rods were carefully withdrawn and the highly radioactive uranium produced the first controlled atomic chain reaction. It ran for only 4.5 minutes at one-half watt but would lead to the technology that made possible the development of the atomic bomb only three years later. Among the small group of scientists present on that historical day was Leo Szilard, a Hungarian theoretical physicist and one of the bomb's principal architects. In 1947 Szilard, who had vigorously opposed the use of the bomb, left physics for biology. He went to Cold Spring Harbor to join the "phage group" of Luria and Delbrück.

Watson's interest, however, had always been in biology. He obtained his degree in 1946, staying on an additional year to take courses in zoology. In 1944 he chanced to read the newly published book by Erwin Schrödinger, *What Is Life?* The book had been inspired by a brief paper written by Max Delbrück on the theoretical physical properties of the gene. Schrodinger speculated further on the nature of the gene in light of the established principles of chemistry and physics. The book's theme is that genes are the key components in living cells and that to understand what life is one must know how genes act. Watson at once "became polarized towards finding out the secret of the gene."

When Watson arrived at the graduate school of Indiana University in 1947, its most prominent faculty member was Herman Muller, who had just won the Nobel prize after his work with X-ray-induced mutations. Although drawn to Indiana by Muller's presence, Watson was most influenced there by Salvadore Luria and through him by Max Delbrück

and the "phage group." Both Luria and Delbrück had fled Europe as war
drew nearer, Luria from Italy and Delbrück from Germany. Luria
assigned Watson to a research project on the effects of X rays on phages
and the latter completed his Ph.D. in May 1950 at the age of 22. After a
last six weeks at Cold Spring Harbor he sailed for Europe.

His experience in Herman Kalckar's lab quickly turned out to be a
disaster. Watson's indifference to nucleic acid chemistry was not cured by
the romance of being in Europe. He became increasingly frustrated by
the growing realization that remaining in Copenhagen with Kalckar
would not get him any closer to the nature of the gene.

Then, while attending a conference in Naples, his fortunes changed.
Among the speakers was Maurice Wilkins from King's College, London.
Wilkins reviewed his preliminary data on the molecular structure of DNA
that he had obtained by the use of X-ray crystallography. Basically, this
technique involves exposing molecules in a crystalline form to X rays.
Some of these rays strike the atoms and are deflected from the crystalline
substance. A rotation of the crystal changes the angles at which the X
rays strike it and the image of the deflected rays can be captured on film.
This "diffraction" pattern can convey information about the three-
dimensional configuration of the atoms making up the molecule.

The technique is precise and demands skilled interpretation for
peering at molecules in a way that nothing else can. Watson had worried
that the structure of genes might be frustratingly irregular. Now he knew
that they could crystallize, that is, they must have a regular structure that
might be analyzed in a systematic way. As Wilkins spoke, Watson
decided to join him in working on DNA in England.

Wilkins, a New Zealand physicist, had come to the United States
during World War II to work on uranium separation for the Manhattan
Project. He soon turned away from the study of the atomic nucleus to
work on the nucleus of the cell, another of the number of physicists who
had decided to turn their skills to understanding biological problems.
Watson, unable to angle an invitation to work directly with Wilkins,
nevertheless managed through Luria's efforts to obtain an invitation to
join Max Perutz's group at the Cavendish Laboratory at Cambridge
University, near King's College.

At that time a concerted effort headed by Perutz was underway to analyze large biological molecules. His group was particularly interested in X-ray crystallography of the hemoglobin protein. The Cavendish was then headed by Sir Lawrence Bragg, one of the inventors of crystallography. It had been the site of the first atom smasher and Ernest Rutherford's original accelerator was still there. Now the Cavendish would be the scene of yet another extraordinary scientific revolution. Rutherford had already unleashed the awesome power locked within the atom. Finally the time had arrived to break open the gene's mysteries to release its potential.

As the inheritor of a past in which Americans dropped nuclear bombs, we can know too well what destruction that triumph of physics wrought on our fellow humans. Physics has also enabled us to glean deep insights into the nature of the universe and of matter. These insights led to extraordinary developments such as computers, supersonic aircraft, rockets, and lasers. These advances, though in themselves morally neutral, can be used either for wise or destructive purposes.

Similarly a new frontier in molecular biology is upon us. We are only now approaching through the Human Genome Project and all of the research that it will inspire an intimate understanding of our genes. This will bring with it a power over human life which must be used wisely. There is much more to be said on this theme in later chapters, so let us return to the drama at hand: the revolutionary discovery of the structure and essence of the gene.

During Watson's first day at Cambridge he met the ebullient Francis Crick and the two hit it off immediately. Not only did they have similar interests but, as Crick would write in his 1988 retrospective *What Mad Pursuit*, "(we had) a certain youthful arrogance, a ruthlessness, and an impatience with sloppy thinking (that) came naturally to both of us." For his part, Watson began his best-selling 1968 book *The Double Helix* with this sentence, "I have never seen Francis Crick in a modest mood."

At that time Francis Crick was 35 years old and was still a graduate student. He was another convert from physics and had joined Perutz at the Cavendish to work on protein structure. Like Watson, Crick had decided early on that only a detailed molecular analysis of DNA would uncover the true nature of the gene. They soon agreed upon a collaboration based on Crick's contributing his knowledge of X-ray crystallography and physics to Watson's familiarity with genetics.

As talented enthusiasts but virtual unknowns in the world of science they had a formidable competitor. Linus Pauling, professor at Cal Tech, was considered the world's leading chemist. He was the author of the classic book *The Nature of the Chemical Bond*, and had only recently described the first protein structure analyzed by X-ray crystallography, calling it an "alpha helix." By this he meant that the particular protein molecule under study existed in a helical shape, that is, a configuration with a constant diameter throughout its length such as a strand of wire would make if it were wrapped around a cylinder.

Pauling's insistence that knowledge of the chemistry of the atoms and bonds of the large molecules of living systems would be sufficient to lay bare the mysteries of living systems had already been an inspiration to both Watson and Crick. It appeared to be only a matter of time before the great Pauling would discover the exact shape of the DNA molecule. With the brashness of youth they determined to beat Pauling at his own game.

To add to their frustration, the work on the DNA molecule at Cambridge now was centered in Maurice Wilkin's laboratory at King's College. In 1950 Sir John Randall, head of the biophysics section at King's, had invited Rosalind Franklin, then working in Paris and a specialist in X-ray analysis of molecules, to come to King's College and set up an X-ray diffraction unit. Wilkins had already done some X-ray analysis of DNA but, knowing he did not have the background to go much further, he had agreed that Randall should hire her to pick up where he had left off. The story of Rosalind Franklin is a complex and dark chapter in the DNA story.

Rosalind Franklin, a bright, analytical, and independent 30-year-old woman, was generally perceived as something of an anomaly in the male club atmosphere of King's College. Shortly after she arrived she began working under the perfectly logical impression that DNA was now her province. She was soon openly annoyed at what she perceived as Wilkins's treatment of her as an assistant rather than as a colleague. The two, as Wilkins so discreetly put it, "never hit it off." The relationship between Wilkins and Franklin and the attendant difficulties that she had to face are carefully and thoughtfully documented in Anne Sayre's book *Rosalind Franklin and DNA*. Arthur Cooper of *Newsweek* said of her book in his review, "Anyone who read 'The Double Helix' owes it to Franklin to read her story too."

Watson's best-seller *The Double Helix*, first published in 1968, is a textbook example of male chauvinism. He referred to Franklin as "Rosy" and wondered "how she would look if she took off her glasses and did something novel with her hair." The epilogue of his book admits that his initial impressions of her "were often wrong" and realized "years too late the struggles that the intelligent woman faces . . ."

Francis Crick, in his retrospective of those years, *What Mad Pursuit*, aproached the subject somewhat differently. He noted that there were "irritating restrictions—she was not allowed to have coffee in one of the faculty rooms reserved for men only—but these were mainly trivial, or so they seemed to be at the time." One cannot imagine their being trivial to the excluded party.

Deprived of any official opportunity to tackle the problem of DNA structure Watson and Crick nevertheless proceeded to emulate Pauling's work on proteins by puzzling over the following question. Based on what they could learn from the X-ray data already gathered by Wilkins and Franklin, they asked themselves which atoms in the DNA molecule were most likely to sit next to which others? All they had to do, according to Watson, with the self-assuredness of hindsight, was to "construct a set of molecular models and begin to play . . ."

In the early 1940s scientists had mistakenly thought that DNA was a small and relatively simple molecule. The leading expert on nucleic acids in the 1920s had been Phoebus Levine of the Rockefeller Institute. He had described the DNA molecule as a regularly repeating series of building blocks called nucleotides, each made of a sugar, phosphate, and nitrogenous base in which the four different types of nucleotides followed one another in fixed order in repeated sets of four. This would form a polymer, a long chain made of many individual building blocks. The "tetra-nucleotide hypothesis," as it was called, left little room for variation in the DNA molecule. This strengthened the case for proteins as the genetic material.

Proteins were known to be definite polymers, whose building blocks were amino acids. These acids are joined to one another like pearls on a string. Twenty different types of amino acids are known to occur commonly in living systems. Unlike the hypothetical monotonous sets of four nucleotide types repeated again and again in nucleic acids, a protein would have many more possibilities for variability. That is because the 20 amino acids could be arranged in literally millions of different sequences. A protein actually consists of one or more individual chains, "polypeptides," usually made up of several hundred amino acids. The polypeptide chains are linked to each other by chemical bonds and the whole complex is contorted into either a roughly spherical or elongated threadlike shape.

X-ray analysis of numerous proteins had shown that each particular protein has a specific unvarying shape particular to that protein type. If heated, some of the protein bonds break apart. The protein literally unfolds, losing its normal precise shape. This is known as "denaturing" the protein. A familiar example of this occurs when egg white, which consists of the protein albumin, is heated. This denaturing changes the egg white from a liquid to a solid form, reflecting the change in the shape in the albumin molecules.

Since scientists found that denatured proteins no longer could function as enzymes, they conjectured that the function of a protein depends on its exact three-dimensional structure. Therefore, if genes were made out of protein, it seemed logical that each gene would have its own unique, three-dimensional organization, just as enzymes did. How could such a complicated structure possibly function as a gene? How could it somehow synthesize other differently shaped proteins to be used as enzymes? For that matter, how could that kind of complex gene copy itself generation after generation with few mistakes?

By the late 1940s several important discoveries clarifying the chemistry of DNA had been made. Scientists had established that DNA molecules were actually quite long and certainly more complex than the unvarying sequence described by Levine. The nucleotide building blocks of DNA each consisted of a sugar (deoxyribose), a phosphate group, and one of four different complex organic molecules termed nitrogenous bases.

Although it is difficult to visualize, we need to understand that molecules take up space in all dimensions. They have specific shapes with constituent atoms attached to each other at a variety of angles. Physical chemists specialize in studying these configurations and have literally worked out three-dimensional scale models for a number of molecules. The internal forces holding molecules together follow certain well-defined physical laws which impose strict constraints on the shape of that molecule.

This means, for example, that a molecule of water or a molecule of glucose can only assume a certain specific shape. However, even if one has a complete analysis of all of the various parts of a highly complex molecule, there are still numerous possible configurations which might seem reasonable to anyone attempting to build a three-dimensional model of that molecule. Given the parts of an automobile transmission, how many ways could they be put together before the engine would operate as designed? Regardless of the possibilities, only one arrangement would be the correct one.

Irwin Chargaff, an Austrian refugee and later a chemist at Columbia University, had made a puzzling discovery in the late 1940s. He found that the composition of DNA from different organisms was quite similar in certain respects. Two of the four nitrogenous base components of DNA, the so-called purines adenine (A) and guanine (G), were made up of two attached rings of atoms, one five-sided and the other six-sided. The rings were made up of carbon, hydrogen, oxygen, and nitrogen. The other two bases were the pyrimidines cytosine (C) and thymine (T), both six-sided rings. Moreover, Chargaff ascertained that the amount of adenine in a given DNA sample always equaled the amount of thymine. Likewise, the amount of guanine equaled that of cytosine. However, there was a critical difference among the DNA isolated from different species of organisms. Although the amount of A equaled that of T and G that of C, the relative amounts of A + T and G + C varied widely. There was no obvious explanation.

The nitrogenous bases, with their relative amounts conforming to what became known as Chargaff's rules, were known to be attached to a long chain of alternating deoxyribose sugar and phosphate groups. One of the four possible nitrogenous bases was bonded to each deoxyribose. A nucleotide consisted of a deoxyribose sugar, phosphate, and nitrogenous base combination.

Watson and Crick could see that the solution to the DNA puzzle was bound to be trickier than that of the alpha helix described by Linus Pauling. In the alpha helix, a single row of attached amino acids coiled up into a helix. The shape was kept intact by "hydrogen bonds" linking together nearby coils of the helical chain. A hydrogen bond forms when a hydrogen atom bound to a negatively charged atom is attracted to another negative atom. In a living cell, these negatively charged atoms are usually oxygen and nitrogen. One hydrogen bond is relatively weak and easily broken but in the case of proteins and other complex molecules there may be many of these bonds and the total attractive force is thus much stronger.

Wilkins's early X-ray data had indicated that the DNA molecule was wider than would be the case if it consisted of only one nucleotide chain. That had led him to the conclusion that DNA was perhaps a compound helix composed of several nucleotide chains wrapped around each other. The chains might be held together by hydrogen bonds or possibly bonds between the phosphate groups.

Watson and Crick began with the assumption that the nucleotides were made up of a "sugar–phosphate backbone," a long unbranched chain of alternating deoxyribose and phosphates. The deoxyribose units of the "backbone" each bore an attached nitrogenous base. The sequence of the nitrogenous bases, each one attached to a molecule of deoxyribose, was assumed to be quite irregular. If the sequence of bases was regular, such as ATGCATGCATGC, then the DNA molecule would be a homogeneous series of nucleotides with nothing to distinguish one gene (whatever that was) from the next. On the other hand, if the order of the bases was irregular, such as AATGCTACT, then this kind of base arrangement could supply incredible variability to the DNA molecule.

What were needed were more definitive X-ray photographs. Rosalind Franklin was scheduled to give a talk on her past-six-months' work and Watson and Crick's attention turned to her latest findings. Watson, who attended the talk with Maurice Wilkins, detailed her remarks to Crick, who seized upon the fact that her current X-ray pictures had been made using hydrated DNA. That meant that the DNA was in the so-called B-form, a descriptive term coined by Franklin, which contained many molecules of water and was thus more fiberlike in nature than the highly crystalline form previously seen by Wilkins. The problem with the presence of so much water was that the clarity of the resulting pictures was poor, making it difficult to interpret. Using Watson's recollection of the amount of water in her samples, Crick determined that DNA could be composed of two, three, or four nucleotide strands. It was "merely" a question of the way in which those strands twisted about the axis.

A few days later a three-membered helix model had been constructed using sheet metal figures cut in the shape and size of the constituent atoms, with wire, nuts, and bolts to hold them together. The nitrogenous bases faced outward and the helix was held together at the center by bonds between the phosphate groups. Proudly showing their construction to Wilkins and Franklin for their approval they were devastated to learn that Watson had misunderstood the amount of water in her sample by a factor of 10.

To make matters worse, the growing tension caused by the proprietary interest that King's College had in DNA and the unofficial efforts with the same by Watson and Crick resulted in official word from above. Sir Lawrence Bragg indicated in no uncertain terms that they would henceforth leave the DNA problem alone. Watson, with his characteristic bravura, wrote about this moratorium, "Lying low made sense because we were up the creek with models based on sugar and phosphate cores." Their active model building was brought to a halt but their conversations and speculations continued unabated.

Meanwhile, Watson had received a long letter from Alfred Hershey at Cold Spring Harbor filled with exciting news about Hershey's latest experiments. He and Martha Chase had established that the key feature of infection of bacteria by viruses was the injection of DNA from the virus into the bacterium. The DNA took over the operations of the bacterial cell, directing it to make new viruses. This was a powerful proof that DNA was the prime genetic material. Not long afterward a chemist from the 'States stopped by the Cavendish for a brief visit. Erwin Chargaff, now one of the world's experts on DNA chemistry, was not amused when he met the two unknowns who proclaimed that they had been in on the race to be the first to understand the three-dimensional structure of DNA. He was doubly taken aback to find that Crick had momentarily forgotten the formulas for the nitrogenous bases. He left unimpressed but Chargaff's rules now entered their calculations. That would prove to be crucial to their success.

One morning a manuscript arrived from the renowned Linus Pauling detailing his conclusions about DNA structure. It was sent to his son Peter who was at that time, ironically, an office mate of Crick and Watson. Their dismay turned to disbelief as they poured over the report and saw that Pauling had made a fundamental error in chemistry. Chemists had long ago established that the phosphate groups of the nucleotides ionized, that is, they released hydrogen into their surroundings. This property of being a "hydrogen donor" made the DNA molecule an acid. Incredibly, Pauling had drawn the phosphate group in the three-membered helix with the hydrogens still attached. The race by no means was over.

Watson rushed to King's College with the Pauling news. He burst in on Rosalind Franklin, working alone in her laboratory. She had long been offended by his continued insistence on lecturing to her on interpreting the X-ray crystallography evidence. According to Watson's accounts, which are the only records of this encounter, as he waved Pauling's manuscript about in his excitement she became angry. Her anger was compounded by the fact that the manuscript he had in his hand contained information which she had only a month before requested unsuccessfully from Pauling's lab.

Watson hastily retreated through the open door whereupon Wilkins appeared and bustled him along to his office. In a spirit of camaraderie, perhaps engendered by their common animosity toward Rosalind Frank-lin, Wilkins showed Watson a picture of an X-ray pattern, one of two excellent pictures of the B-form of DNA that Franklin had taken ten months earlier. Watson wrote of the experience, "The instant I saw the picture my mouth fell open and my pulse began to race."

He had the new critical facts that were needed. The B-form of DNA was a helix which had a regular repeating interval of 34 angstroms distance between each coil. An angstrom is one ten-billionth of a meter; there are 254 million angstrom units to one inch. This was precisely 10 times the 3.4 angstrom distance between one nucleotide and the next one above it. The helix itself was a smooth cylinder 20 angstroms wide.

Watson had already been aware of some of these measurements.

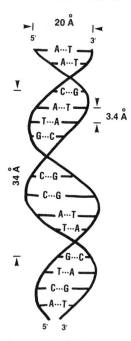

The double helix of DNA. The two winding lines represent the sugar–phosphate chains. Note that their antiparallel arrangement is indicated by a 5′ and a 3′ at opposite ends. See Chapter 5 for further details.

Whether or not Wilkins discussed the others at that time is still unclear. The fact remains that he showed Watson the picture without the knowledge of Rosalind Franklin. She already had deduced that the nitrogenous bases had to be in the center of the helix with the sugar phosphate backbone on the outside. Her own notes say that "the results suggest a helical structure . . . containing 2, 3 or 4 co-axial nucleic acid chains per helical unit, and having the phosphate groups near the outside." Wilkins had shown Watson the very photograph by Rosalind Franklin that would be crucial to building a correct molecular model.

On hearing of the Pauling fiasco and convinced that Watson and

Crick, now armed with their new information, were prepared to complete their synthesis, Bragg gave them renewed permission to resume model building. Days of frustration followed. One month after Watson's viewing of the B-form of DNA in Wilkins's lab a report was passed on to Crick which had been circulated by Sir John Randall. It contained a report by Rosalind Franklin giving the critical measurements of the B-form but not the photograph. Crick, with a much deeper understanding than Watson of X-ray crystallography gleaned from her numbers the last piece of the puzzle.

Crick suggested that the sugar–phosphate backbones of the double helix would have to be realigned so that they ran in opposite directions to each other, a so-called antiparallel fashion. This orientation was necessary in order that the two sides of the helix, joined together by the base pairs, would conform to the known 20-angstrom diameter.

Armed with this new realization, Watson redoubled his efforts. The "eureka" moment arrived. He suddenly realized that an adenine and thymine pair when held tightly by two hydrogen bonds would be identical in size to a guanine and cytosine pair held together by three such bonds. Chargaff's rules! If these AT and GC pairs were placed into a double helix model made of two intertwining sugar–phosphate backbones so that the base pairs lay flat, their dimensions would allow precisely ten base pairs to fit into every 34-angstrom complete turn of the helical coils. In so doing, each flat base pair was not aligned with the one immediately above and below it, but was slightly offset from the next like the stairs in a winding staircase. Each was rotated 36 degrees with respect to the adjacent pair. Everything fit.

This pairing fit the configuration of two backbones of sugar phosphate units joined to each other by these pairs of nitrogenous bases. The double helix was "right-handed." If one could look down its longitudinal axis, the two sugar–phosphate backbones would turn counterclockwise as they approached the viewer. The model was complete. According to Watson, "It was too pretty not to be true."

A 900-word article by James Watson and Francis Crick was sent off on April 2, 1953 to the editors of *Nature*, a leading international science journal. It began modestly: "We wish to suggest a structure for . . . DNA. This structure has novel features which are of considerable interest." The "novel features" of the molecule would include the gene itself.

"This structure," whose analysis had long been the province of chemists, joined later by X-ray crystallographers, had in the end been uncovered by two creative minds not among their ranks. They had used neither test tubes, incubators, nor chemicals—only the sheer intellectual power of synthesis. A significant part of the data which had entered into their synthesis had been derived by Rosalind Franklin. She had taken the definitive X-ray photograph, and her calculations were vital in the formation of the final model. Would she have eventually come up with the answer herself? Very likely.

However, she would not be chosen to share the glory with Watson, Crick, and Wilkins, who received the Nobel prize in 1962—not even posthumously. Rosalind Franklin died of cancer in 1958 at the age of 37. According to Watson, she "continued working on a high level until a few weeks before her death."

Our treatment of the search for the gene from the days of Mendel to the era of Watson and Crick has been necessarily brief. We have developed only an outline of the progressively numerous and important developments which culminated in the publication of the elegant model of DNA. This marvelous synthesis captured the attention of the scientific world.

However, despite the fact that the beautifully symmetrical intricacies of the DNA molecule had at last been laid bare, the gene itself remained undefined, hidden somewhere in that complex molecule. It would not remain so for long, as experiments proliferated based upon the newly clarified image of DNA.

Meanwhile, a second paper by Watson and Crick, "The Genetic Implications of the Structure of Deoxyribonucleic Acid" appeared one month later. They suggested that during cell division DNA (and thereby the chromosomes) copies itself following a separation of the two sides of the helix caused by a breaking of the hydrogen bonds between the bases. This would leave each of the two nucleotide strands as a template for forming a complementary nucleotide strand. That is, each nitrogenous base would be exposed (unpaired) and a new nucleotide with compatible nitrogenous bases (A with T, G with C) would form on each of these. The original and the new strand would then reform the helical configuration and the result would be two double helices and hence two chromosomes where there had been one.

All of this was purely speculative. They admitted that there was no evidence for how the helices could unwind and separate or how new nucleotides could form and join to the original. At this point they were not even sure that the chromosome was one long DNA chain, admitting the possibility that it could be "patches of the acid joined together by protein."

Logical explanations without proof bear little weight in science but often form an important framework for experimentation. Such was the case with Watson and Crick's schema.

In 1957, Matthew Meselson, a graduate student in Linus Pauling's lab at Cal Tech, along with a postdoctoral fellow, Franklin Stahl, devised an ingenious approach to this problem of DNA replication. They hit upon the notion of tracking the course of replication by labeling the DNA molecule, not by radioactivity, as in the phage experiment by Hershey and Chase, but by using isotopes.

An isotope is an alternate form of a chemical element which differs from other atoms of the same element in the number of neutrons in the nucleus. This makes the isotope form slightly "heavier," that is, different in atomic weight. Fortunately a nonradioactive isotope of nitrogen had only recently been made commercially available, the so-called heavy form of nitrogen, ^{15}N. Meselson and Stahl grew a dense population of many generations of *E. coli* bacteria in a food source rich with the isotope, thus ensuring that the heavy nitrogen would be picked up by the bacteria and incorporated into all of the nitrogenous bases of the bacterial DNA. Keeping a sample of this culture, they immediately transferred the remaining bacteria to a food source containing ordinary nitrogen, ^{14}N. As new generations of bacteria formed, they were removed for analysis.

Spun down in a centrifuge, the bacteria formed a pellet at the bottom of the centrifuge tube. The bacterial cells were then broken open, releasing the cell contents. A sample of these cell contents was placed into a centrifuge tube filled with a solution of cesium chloride. This is a substance which they had found would form a gradient of concentration in a tube when spun at high speeds. That is, the upper level of the tube would become dilute and the concentration would gradually increase toward the bottom where the densest concentration of the cesium chloride would be located. Molecules placed in this gradient and centrifuged would end up suspended at a concentration level which would support their particular weight.

The DNA from the first sample, removed before the normal nitrogen was introduced and which therefore was filled with the heavy isotope, formed a sharp band toward the lower, denser end of the gradient. On the other hand, the band from an untreated bacterial culture containing no isotope was much further up in the tube.

DNA from the cells grown for one generation, that is, after one chromosome replication, formed a band between the two. This meant that they were somewhat lighter than the isotope-laden DNA and heavier than the untreated sample. After two generations (two chromosome replications) two bands formed, one identical to that of the first generation and another lighter band matching the level of the band of untreated DNA.

This brief, ingenious experiment offered clear proof that the replication of DNA occurred exactly as Watson and Crick had predicted. The double helix containing heavy nitrogen had come apart and new nucleotides containing normal nitrogen formed a new complementary strand. In the first generation, therefore, all of the DNA in the double helix consisted of one strand of the original DNA molecule and a new unlabeled strand. In the next generation, those half-labeled double helices would open up and replicate, resulting in an equal mixture of totally unlabeled DNA helices and half-labeled DNA helices.

The young students had given biological confirmation of the double helix and its copying mechanism. In addition, their cesium chloride density gradient method, which they had concocted during an evening conversation over their dinner table, is now a universal technique for extracting and separating large quantities of DNA.

By the early 1950s, though evidence had begun to point to genetic control as somehow involving the regulation of how cells make proteins, it was unclear whether or not any of this protein building actually

(a)	(b)	(c)
G – C	G – c	g – C
T – A	T – a	t – A
T – A	T – a	t – A
A – G	A – g	a – G
G – C	G – c	g – C
G – C	G – c	g – C
A – T	A – t	a – T
T – A	T – a	t – A

(a) In replication, this double helix splits apart at the bonds between the nitrogenous bases. (b,c) Each side of the original double helix acts as a template for the formation of a new complementary strand. The new bases are indicated here as lower-case letters. Only the nitrogenous bases of the DNA nucleotides are shown.

occurred in the nucleus itself. Most evidence pointed to the cytoplasm, that area surrounding the nucleus, as the site of protein manufacture. This would require some intermediate between the DNA in the nuclear chromosomes and the cytoplasm. A prime candidate for that "messenger" would eventually be another nucleic acid, RNA, or "ribonucleic acid."

As far back as the 1920s, nucleic acids were known to be of two types. The most abundant was DNA, deoxyribonucleic acid which, along with some protein, forms the chromosomes. The other was RNA, ribonucleic acid, present in smaller amounts in cells. RNA is chemically different from DNA in that RNA contains the sugar ribose rather than deoxyribose and the nitrogenous base uracil rather than thymine.

After 1953 Watson turned his attention to RNA as the other nucleic acid left to be analyzed. At Cal Tech he began working on X-ray analysis of RNA. It proved immensely frustrating, for RNA could not be crystallized. RNA would not readily yield its secrets by the same tactics that had uncovered DNA structure.

Meanwhile, the electron microscope had been improved to the point where one could begin to see extraordinary cell detail. Studies of the supposedly formless cytoplasm of plants and animals were beginning to reveal an amazingly intricate network of membranous channels continuous with the nuclear membrane. Scattered along the outer surface of these channels were thousands of small, roughly spherical particles, later named "ribosomes." They were made of protein and RNA. In 1953 George Palade of the Rockefeller Institute showed that these abundant particles were also found in bacterial cells, though not associated with any network.

Also in 1953 (a most productive year in the history of biology), Paul Zamecnik, a physician–researcher at Massachusetts General Hospital, inserted a key piece into the puzzle. Using amino acids containing a radioactive isotope of carbon, ^{14}C, he traced the site of protein synthesis in rat liver cells to those very same ribosomal particles. Zamecnik went on to develop a technique whereby liver cells could be ground up and the resulting organic soup centrifuged, leaving a liquid suspension of cellular components now liberated from the cells.

This "cell-free" system could be further purified and used as a medium for examining protein synthesis in great detail. Amino acids could be added singly and in various combinations. Nucleic acids could be introduced and isotopes traced to follow the path of the various ingredients. This would prove to be a key technique for unlocking the genetic code.

During his months of puzzling over the DNA model, Watson had pasted to his wall a statement which read, "DNA to RNA to protein." He postulated that "information" from DNA was somehow "passed on" by RNA to regulate the sequence of the amino acids in a protein. The DNA molecule consisted of an unpredictable mixed sequence of nitrogenous bases which were joined across the center of the double helix by hydrogen bonds. This had immediately suggested several possibilities to Watson and Crick concerning the nature of the role of chromosomes in protein synthesis as well as their replication during cell division.

Crick wanted to speculate at length about these ideas in the original 1953 *Nature* paper but agreed to postpone discussion about protein synthesis and insert only the simple statement, "It has not escaped our notice that the specific pairing we have postulated immediately suggests a possible copying mechanism for the genetic material."

This seems to us now to be a classical understatement. Scientists are accustomed to what seems to be a perfectly logical story of DNA replication and genetic function. However, their understanding was by no means at all clear in those early days. For example, Alfred Hershey wrote in 1953 that DNA would "not prove to be a unique determinant of genetic specificity"!

A growing number of laboratories began to search for whatever intermediates there might be between DNA and proteins. This line of inquiry quickly became broad and complex and for our purposes is best summarized as follows.

By the end of 1956, biochemists using cell-free extracts and bacterial systems had put together a sketchy outline of protein synthesis which included RNA as a "carrier" molecule. This meant that it apparently picked up amino acids and brought them to the ribosomes. Each amino acid appeared to have its own specific RNA molecule and the attachment of the amino acid to the RNA was accomplished by specific enzymes. It was as though there had to be 20 different workers, each bringing a separate part to an assembly line.

Over the next several years important details filled out this picture. Zamecnik's lab discovered that every one of these carrier RNAs had the same nucleotide sequence on one end of the molecule. It was a row of three nucleotides that had the nitrogen base sequence cytosine–cytosine–adenine (CCA). The amino acid became attached at that three-base site. This type of RNA, which carried the amino acids, became known as "transfer RNA," or tRNA, because it apparently transferred the amino acids from the cytoplasm to the ribosome.

Robert Holley, a biochemist at the New York State Agricultural Experiment Station at Cornell, completed the gargantuan task over a seven-year period, of determining the exact sequence of nitrogenous bases in a transfer RNA molecule. It turned out to be 77 nucleotides long and had a peculiar cloverleaf shape. At one end of the chain of nucleotides was the CCA sequence for amino acid attachment. At the far end was a segment that proved to be a key element in the process of protein synthesis. It was a three-nucleotide sequence that contained three nitrogenous bases complementary to a set of bases located on the ribosome.

Finally, also in the late 1950s, François Jacob and Jacques Monod at the Institut Pasteur in Paris traced a complex series of cellular events in bacteria which almost completed the picture. Their results showed that there was a second form of RNA involved which acted as an intermediate between DNA and the ribosome. They christened it "messenger RNA," or mRNA. Unlike transfer RNA, messenger RNA is a long, straight-chain molecule.

By 1960 the evidence accumulated from diverse sources pointed to a scenario for gene function. A gene in the DNA transfers information to a messenger RNA which carries that message to a ribosome. Molecules of transfer RNA then bring amino acids to the ribosome and the correct sequence of amino acids to make the protein is stitched together following the information in the messenger RNA. What information would a gene have to contain if its role were, in fact, to direct the formation of a protein? And how could that message be passed on to a messenger RNA molecule? What was the relationship between transfer RNA and this messenger?

In that amazingly fruitful year of 1953, the English biochemist Fred Sanger, working at the Cavendish Laboratory, had laid the groundwork for clarifying those issues. He announced that after a decade of painstaking work he had become the first to trace the complete sequence of amino acids in a protein. He had analyzed insulin, which had turned out to be a small protein consisting of two amino acid chains (polypeptides), one with 30 amino acids and the other with 21.

From classical biochemistry had come an extraordinarily timely and critical step in developing a frame of reference for the analysis of the genetic code of DNA. The amino acids sequence in a protein was specific and consistent which suggested strongly that it was determined by a "code": some set of instructions operative during the assemblage of these building blocks into the same sequence time after time. Sanger's pioneering work was followed in 1956 by Vernon Ingram's analysis of yet another protein.

Ingram was a biochemist who had worked on protein chemistry at the Rockefeller Institute before joining Max Perutz's group at the Cavendish. Crick, realizing that proof was needed for his hypothesis that a mutant gene would probably produce a change in the amino acid sequence of a protein, had convinced Ingram to tackle the problem with him. Because of the long-standing interest in the hemoglobin molecule,

Perutz's lab was well supplied with hemoglobin in both normal and abnormal forms. The abnormal hemoglobin had been isolated from the blood of patients with sickle-cell anemia, a severe and ultimately fatal hereditary disease that affects African and American blacks.

Perutz had tried to distinguish between the two forms of hemoglobin by X-ray crystallography but to no avail. In the disease, when oxygen levels in the blood lower, as in exertion, the red blood cells containing the oxygen-carrying hemoglobin become misshapen into elongated, twisted arcs fancifully likened to the shape of a sickle. These weakened cells readily burst as they squeeze through tiny blood capillaries. Anemia, fatigue, and a lowered resistance to infection result. The incidence of this disease is high; about 2 in every 1000 American blacks suffer from the disease.

Eighty in every 1000 black persons studied have red cells that will only form these sickle shapes at very low oxygen concentrations. They are "carriers," for while they themselves do not suffer the pains of the disease, if both mother and father are carriers, their children are at risk. The odds of their child inheriting sickle-cell anemia are one out of four. In genetic terms, that means that a dominant gene for normal hemoglobin is present on each one of a pair of chromosomes in the normal parent's cells. However, carriers have one dominant and one recessive mutant gene. A chance combination of two recessive mutant genes in the offspring of two carriers will result in the disease.

In the late 1940s Linus Pauling and one of his students, Harvey Itano, had demonstrated that a slight difference existed between normal and sickle-cell cell hemoglobins. He used the technique of "electrophoresis" in which a solution of the two hemoglobins was exposed to an electric current. The normal hemoglobin migrated toward the positive pole and the sickle-cell hemoglobin toward the negative pole, indicating a slight charge difference and thus a small variation in chemical structure between the two molecules. Efforts to determine the exact nature of this variation had failed until Ingram's ingenious analysis.

Ingram cut up the hemoglobin protein, known to be two connected polypeptide chains, into smaller segments called peptides. He used an enzyme which cuts between specific amino acids resulting in fragments about ten amino acids in length. Utilizing Sanger's effective but piecemeal techniques to analyze the fragments would have taken years. Ingram devised a rapid method to look for differences along the fragments. He first applied his digested sample to a piece of moist filter paper and used electrophoresis to achieve partial separation of the peptides. He followed this with "paper chromatography" in which an edge of the filter paper containing the partially separated peptides is placed into a chemical solvent. As the solvent slowly migrates up the paper, just as a paper towel absorbs a spill, it carries the peptides with it. Depending on how soluble they are, the peptides periodically leave the solvent and cling to the filter paper at different sites.

The resulting consistently reproducible pattern formed by electrophoresis in one direction, followed by paper chromatography at right angles to the first, showed that there was indeed one slightly positively charged piece in the sickle-cell hemoglobin not found in the normal form. Ingram called this chromatographic pattern the "fingerprint" of the protein. Modifications of his technique bearing this name are today universally used in the separation of complex mixtures, including DNA fragments, a procedure essential to the Human Genome Project.

Ingram's further analysis confirmed that the devastating disease of sickle-cell anemia is caused merely by the presence of one incorrect amino acid in one of the four polypeptide chains of hemoglobin. With Ingram's brilliant work, the concept of the unit of heredity passed beyond speculation into experimental demonstration. He had confirmed that this basic unit should be seen as something which was a code for determining the correct position of a specific amino acid within the sequence of amino acids making up a protein.

A rapid screening test is now available and is widely used to determine the presence of the "sickling trait" in carriers. This information can be used in counseling potential parents on the risks for their children. The pattern of inheritance of this condition was confirmed in 1949. Diagnostic procedures for other important genetic disorders have since been developed but relatively few compared to what will be possible with our expanding analysis of the human genome. New detailed information already being discovered about some of the many thousands of genes within the human genome will make possible highly refined genetic analyses, many of which will serve, like the sickling trait test, as the basis for predicting risk factors. (The consequences and controversies that this raises will be discussed in Chapters 8–11.)

In September of 1957 Francis Crick addressed the Symposium of the Society for Experimental Biology, meeting that year in Cambridge. He had been invited to speak about the synthesis of proteins. Crick had proven to be an intellectual leader in those formative years of molecular biology. In his talk he brilliantly drew together the increasingly confusing maze of data and conjecture about the gene and its function. His bold assertions, most of which have since been proven to be correct, gave a sharp focus to the search that literally pointed the way to discoveries soon to follow.

Crick argued that the main function of the gene is to control the synthesis of proteins. He reviewed the evidence of Sanger that proteins were amino acid chains whose sequence was varied but which was consistent within the same type of protein in a species. He pointed to the experiments of Ingram with sickle-cell anemia and that of other investigators relative to the possible role of RNA and ribosomes. He concluded with a statement of two general principles which he called the *Sequence Hypothesis* and the *Central Dogma*.

The former held that the order in which amino acids appear in protein molecules is determined by a simple "code" consisting of a sequence of nitrogenous bases in a particular section of DNA in a chromosome. The Central Dogma was summarized by Crick as follows: "Once information has passed into protein it cannot get out again." By that he meant that there could be a transfer of information from DNA to RNA or from RNA to protein but never the other way around. By "information" he meant the precise sequence of the nitrogenous bases in the DNA.

Crick's choice of the word "dogma" was not a call for blind faith in this interpretation of the data. According to Horace Judson in his book *The Eighth Day of Creation*, it was based on his erroneous and seemingly cynical definition for that term, that is, "an idea for which there was no reasonable evidence." Crick told Judson "I just didn't know what dogma meant . . . dogma was just a catch phrase."

In the two years following Crick's talk, confusion reigned in the attempts to define the details of the "code." In 1959, according to Crick, "the whole business of the code was a complete mess . . . nothing fitted." Nevertheless, within two years it was solved.

As was so often the case, Francis Crick was central to the solution. He had argued for several years that, assuming the nitrogenous base sequence of DNA nucleotides directed the assembly of amino acids into a chain, that sequence in itself would be sufficient to form the complex protein. Given the correct sequence, the protein could then fold up into its three-dimensional configuration. He had also asserted that the DNA code would be found to be universal, that is, it would be the same in all living organisms. This assumed that such a successful, complicated system had evolved early in the history of living forms and was retained. Like many of Crick's ideas, this was ultimately proven to be essentially correct.

This "genetic code" as Crick termed it most likely consisted of a series of sets of information in DNA, each corresponding to a code for a particular amino acid. With only four possible nitrogenous bases and 20 amino acids, he pointed out that it was obvious that a set of only two nucleotides was limited to only 16 possible combinations. However, a series of three nucleotides would be sufficient for 64 different combinations, more than enough to supply a code for 20 amino acids.

Although laboratories on both sides of the Atlantic had joined in the fray, a small nucleus of scientists including Crick, Watson, Brenner, Meselson, and others had coalesced into what amounted to an "old boy" network. They successfully dazzled first each other and then the rest of the scientific community with their achievements. They visited each other's laboratories, collaborating and communicating there and at the frequent national and international meetings. There was even an RNA tie club, founded half in jest, whose charter was "to solve the riddle of the RNA structure and to understand the way it built proteins." The membership grew to 20, one for each of the amino acids.

While at the International Biochemistry Congress held in Moscow in August, 1961, Matthew Meselson and Walter Gilbert stopped by a small conference room to listen to a talk by a Marshall Warren Nirenberg. This 34-year-old scientist on the staff of the National Institutes of Health (NIH) near Washington, D.C., had apparently done some work with protein synthesis. As he spoke, Meselson and Gilbert were astonished. Meselson alerted Crick who quickly added Nirenberg to the panel of speakers slated to address all of the several hundreds of scientists who had attended the meeting. The second reading of his paper before a packed hall "electrified the audience." This virtual unknown, working quietly with his colleague Johann Matthei, had broken the genetic code.

Marshall Nirenberg's aim in science had been to discover how information flowed from DNA into proteins. When he started on his own in 1959, messenger RNA had not yet been discovered. Nirenberg reasoned that the way to get clear evidence was to set up an experimental system to which he could add nucleic acids and other substances to see how they affected protein synthesis.

With the assistance of Johann Matthei, at NIH from Bonn on a postdoctoral research fellowship, he promptly borrowed Paul Zamecnik's recently published cell-free system, utilizing in this case his newest approach which used *E. coli* rather than rat liver. Into the mix went amino acids that were radioactively labeled so they could be detected. They promptly showed up as parts of newly made proteins. When they added an enzyme that specifically destroys RNA, protein synthesis quickly stopped. Addition of an enzyme that breaks down DNA did not stop the synthesis until about 30 minutes had gone by.

They interpreted this as indicative of a process in which RNA must have acted as an intermediate between DNA and protein synthesis. Destruction of RNA would grind the protein-making machinery to a halt, whereas losing DNA would affect it only when supplies of information in RNA had run out and no new RNA could be made. Without realizing it they had finally demonstrated and confirmed the existence of messenger RNA. At the time of their discovery they did not know that the existence of such a molecule had been postulated by Jacob and Monod shortly before.

Providentially, the chief of their laboratory was Leon Heppel who was skillful in making artificial RNA of different definite composition. Heppel had accumulated a library of such RNAs. On May 22, 1961, Matthei decided to try some of the synthetic RNA. To a solution of RNA made to contain only uracil as its nitrogenous base component he carefully introduced different radioactive amino acids one at a time. Nothing happened until he added the amino acid phenylalanine. The mixture quickly yielded a polypeptide (a chain of amino acids) made entirely of phenylalanine units. The signal, or code, for positioning the amino acid phenylalanine in a polypeptide was repeating units of uracil!

The gene was at hand. After the presentation Meselson ran up to Nirenberg and embraced him.

But were these nitrogenous bases read in a simple series, one after the other? Or was there punctuation, such as a nonused nitrogenous base between the sites of the actual codes? How many nitrogenous bases constituted one unit of the code? For example, did it take three or four or more uracil bases to determine the position of phenylalanine?

Following the Moscow meetings, using bacteriophage and *E. coli*, Crick, Sydney Brenner, and Leslie Barnett finally established the specifics of the genetic code in that same year. They confirmed that it was always a sequence of exactly three nitrogenous bases, "a triplet code," thus confirming an earlier hypothesis of Francis Crick. Three successive nitrogenous bases in the messenger RNA would be the signal for positioning one amino acid in a protein. Each polypeptide formed in Nirenberg's experiments must have been coded in the RNA by three uracils for each phenylalanine. If his synthetic RNA had been the naturally occurring molecule messenger RNA, the code would have existed originally in the DNA. There, three nucleotides containing adenine could act as a code whose instructions would be translated into a messenger RNA with three uracils, since the latter are complementary to adenine.

This finally established that the information transfer in protein synthesis begins with units of three successive nitrogenous bases in the DNA. The information passes from DNA to messenger RNA as the latter is synthesized in the nucleus. The messenger RNA thus carries a code as a base sequence that at the ribosomes is "translated" as a corresponding amino acid sequence.

The gene had been found at last. It is a sequence of nitrogenous bases in the DNA molecule that codes for the synthesis of a polypeptide. Proteins consist of one or more polypeptides.

The practical difficulties of determining which particular sequence coded for which amino acid appeared to be more arduous than it turned

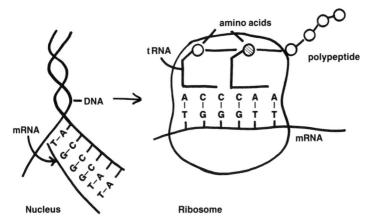

Messenger RNA is made according to the code in DNA. It goes to the ribosome, to which each transfer RNA brings a different amino acid. These are joined together to form a polypeptide according to the message in the messenger RNA sequence.

out to be. That same year a breakthrough occurred that would make such a task feasible. Nirenberg, along with Phillip Leder, a postdoctoral student in his lab, had managed to form lengths of RNA only three nucleotides long which were sufficient to code for one amino acid. Meanwhile, Har Gobind Khorana at the University of Wisconsin had perfected the detailed biochemistry to make long stretches of RNA with known, simple repeating sequences.

Thanks to the methods of Nirenberg and Khorana, by the time of the Cold Spring Harbor Symposium of 1966 the details of genetic code were almost completely solved. Crick proposed what has since become a standard form in which to present the genetic code, listing the sets of three nitrogenous bases on the messenger RNA as "codons." There is more than one codon for most of the amino acids. Three of the 64 codons do not specify amino acids but indicate "stop." One is a "start" codon. These are, in effect, punctuation whose presence translates into "start" or "stop" protein synthesis.

The scheme of protein synthesis could now be outlined as follows. The double helix opens up at a particular site by a breaking of hydrogen bonds. A messenger RNA (mRNA) is synthesized at that opened portion of the helix and the nitrogenous bases of that RNA are complementary to the sequence of bases on one side of the helix. This mRNA goes to the ribosome and becomes attached to it.

A transfer RNA (tRNA) carrying an amino acid attaches to a start codon on the mRNA, now attached to the ribosomes. The linking up of amino acids begins as more tRNAs bring amino acids to the ribosomal–mRNA complex. These tRNAs attach momentarily to the mRNA site where the codon is complementary to a specific set of three bases on the tRNA strand. The ribosome literally moves down the mRNA strand and the successive amino acids are joined to each other one at a time by enzymes. The synthesis ends at a stop codon. The polypeptide strand is released and assumes its final complex shape. In many proteins several polypeptide chains join to form the complete protein molecule.

The details of the crucial role of the genes were finally known. The nitrogenous base codes direct the formation of the cell's proteins. Many of those proteins are the enzymes that drive the chemical reactions of the living cell. Whatever cells and the organisms which they form can do is determined by the genetic codes in those cells.

The "unknown" Marshall Nirenberg, Hans Khorana, and Robert Holley shared the Nobel prize in 1968.

*   *   *

The genome of any organism could from then on be understood in a detailed way undreamt of 20 years earlier. It had been revealed as the full complement of instructions embodied in a series of sets of three DNA nitrogenous bases. The totality of these long sequences were the instructions for the construction, maintenance, and functioning of every living cell. The genome was a dictionary of code words, now translated, that determined what the organism could do. It was the control center of the cell.

Differences among organisms were the result of differences among parts of these genome sequences. During evolution, differences among species could result from changes in the sequences, termed mutations, followed by natural selection. The sequence of amino acids in some proteins and that of the nitrogenous bases in the nucleotides of some RNA molecules had actually been analyzed by scientists. If one could find out the sequence of nitrogenous bases in an organism's DNA, one would know its genetic code.

The average DNA molecule in a human cell is about 140 million nucleotide pairs long. Because atoms are so small, if this molecule were stretched, it would be about 5 centimeters long. The 46 DNA molecules in each cell would total over 2 meters—about 6 feet. Despite the incredible advances that had finally led to an understanding of what the gene actually was, any attempt to determine the sequence of all of the nitrogenous bases within the nucleotides of any complete genome, let alone that of the human, would have been preposterous.

Within a decade, it would no longer be unthinkable. Molecular biology opened yet another chapter which would see the gene, so recently an enigma, become an entity which could be isolated, reproduced in the laboratory, and moved from one organism to another. Science had entered the era of genetic engineering.

5

STICKY ENDS AND A NEW CREATION

James Watson in his book *Recombinant DNA—A Short Course* recalls that in 1966 despite the fact that the genetic code had been fully deciphered molecular biology appeared to some to be at an impasse. Unless some radically new methods emerged to enable scientists to isolate and study individual genes, there appeared to be little prospect of further dramatic advances. According to Watson, to avoid "marking time" several eminent researchers actually left molecular genetics for neurobiology. He was undoubtedly referring to, among others, Francis Crick, who moved on to the field of developmental biology and to the study of the brain.

Crick felt that the foundations of molecular biology had been well established and there remained the lengthy task of "filling in the many details." He did not and could not have foreseen that a veritable avalanche of discoveries would soon sweep through the scientific community and begin a period of excitement and achievement that has had few parallels in the history of biological research.

As has been true of so many other advances in the life sciences, these dramatic breakthroughs arose not as the result of a major organized research program with assigned responsibilities but out of the voluntary study in independent laboratories of seemingly innocuous, and to the nonscientist, perhaps rather insignificant creatures. Some critics, in fact, find fault with the Human Genome Project on the grounds that it is too goal-oriented and might distract individuals and funding from other vital less-showy areas—but more of that discussion later.

The history of science is a rich mosaic of individual lines of inquiry often with no apparent end beyond knowledge of and for itself. Certainly, trends are followed and one conclusion may often advance the search for yet another. Isolated observations, speculations, and seemingly unrelated data may often as not fade into obscurity. They may, however, resurface at precisely the moment needed to further an area perhaps never envisioned by the original investigators. Such was the case once again in molecular biology during the late 1960s as disparate discoveries converged and the brief sense of stasis passed quickly into the realization of unprecedented opportunity.

You will recall our recounting of the discovery of viruses including the bacteriophages, or "phages," the viruses that attack bacteria. The most intensively studied of these had been the phages which infect *Escherichia coli*, more conveniently called *E. coli*. This humble bacterium, first isolated from the feces of an infant in 1888 by Dr. Theodore Escherich, might seem to lack the panache to become a famous player in the drama of genetic history. In fact, with the exception of the human organism, this blunt, rod-shaped cell, less than 1 micrometer (39 millionths of an inch) in length, has been studied more intensively than any other living organism. *E. coli* is our constant companion. It lives in the hundreds of billions in our large intestines in the company of 400 or so other bacterial species. These bacteria are a threat to us only because of the possibility of a life-threatening infection resulting from trauma, puncture of the intestine and release of its contents into the normally sterile abdominal cavity. The important function of these bacteria is to protect against the invasion of disease-causing organisms into the intestinal contents. Such interlopers are routinely overwhelmed by these "friendly" bacteria.

The bacteriophages designated T-even phages are viruses containing DNA that infect *E. coli*. Remember that viruses are not living organisms, but rather are nucleic acids, either DNA or RNA, wrapped in protein. They can propagate themselves only by entering a living cell and utilizing the cellular metabolism to make copies of themselves. They are strange, lifeless parasites which pass from cell to cell, eventually perishing, if one may use that term, if they cannot find and enter a cell and force the cell to do their bidding. Rendering cells inhospitable to harmful viruses is the rationale behind many vaccines.

A dramatic example is that of the smallpox virus vaccine. As the result of a worldwide effort to eradicate smallpox, a viral disease that over the centuries has killed and disfigured millions, the World Health Organization mounted a massive effort to identify and vaccinate all persons in contact with every known smallpox patient. Humans are the only known host for this virus. In October 1975 the last case of smallpox in the world was reported. The virus could no longer find cells without adequate defense mechanisms and the scourge of smallpox disappeared from the planet. The isolation of genes during the Human Genome Project is expected to result in the development of many vaccines otherwise unattainable by conventional methods, to stamp out other pernicious viruses.

By the mid-1960s the rapid breakdown of DNA as well as RNA in solutions made by grinding up of cells in the laboratory was a familiar phenomenon. The destruction of these nucleic acids was traced to "nucleases," enzymes which had been found to exist in many types of cells. These enzymes cleaved the nucleic acids into many random fragments. However, the means by which a cell might rejoin DNA fragments was unknown. Then, in 1967 an enzyme was found which could do just that. Amazingly, this enzyme, DNA ligase, was discovered almost simultaneously by five research groups working independently in separate laboratories.

Before we proceed, it will be useful to review and elaborate on a few details of DNA structure that need to be clearly understood. Let us visualize the DNA double helix simply as a ladder. A ladder has two sidepieces and rungs. The rungs in this analogy are two joined sections, each a complementary pair of nitrogenous bases, either AT or GC. The sidepieces are the deoxyribose sugar (S) and phosphate (P) "backbones" of the helix: they are a continuous strand of S–P–S–P–S–P, and so on. According to chemical protocol, the five carbons of the deoxyribose sugar are numbered to distinguish one from another. In this scheme, they are listed as carbon atoms 1' to 5'. The 5' carbon atom projects from the rest of the ring-shaped sugar molecule. A hydroxyl group (OH) is connected to the 3' carbon.

To continue the ladder analogy, one can say that the left sidepiece

```
S P S P S P S P S P S P S P S
A   T   G   C   T   A   T   C
|   |   |   |   |   |   |   |
T   A   C   G   A   T   A   G
S P S P S P S P S P S P S P S
```

The two sides of the double helix are alternating sugar (S) and phosphate (P)
groups joined to each other. The sides are held together by hydrogen bonds
between pairs of nitrogenous bases (A–T or G–C) which are bonded to the
sugars.

runs from top to bottom and the right sidepiece from the bottom to the
top. The result is that the left sidepiece ends at the top with a phosphate
group projecting from the 5′ carbon atom, and at the bottom with a
hydroxyl group projecting from the 3′ carbon atom. The right sidepiece
is just the opposite. The practical consequences for the molecule are that
this orientation allows it to maintain its symmetrical double helix shape
and function normally. Bear this structure in mind as we continue with
our history.

In 1970, a group working in the laboratory of Har Gobind Khorana,
then at the University of Wisconsin, found that an enzyme DNA ligase
made by *E. coli* could randomly stitch together end to end completely
separated DNA pieces. The reaction was inefficient, since it depended on
ends of the strands coming in direct contact with each other. In order to
render the process more efficient, a way would be needed to hold the two
ends together so the ligase could act.

Such a method was quickly devised at Stanford in both the laboratory of Peter Lobban and A. Dale Kaiser as well as that of David Jackson,
Robert Simons, and Paul Berg. The former group used DNA ligase to
join pieces of cut-up bacteriophage DNA. The latter scientists used the
new technique to join bacteriophage DNA to DNA from an animal virus.

This procedure involved the following basic steps. The DNA was
first treated with an enzyme made by the bacterial phage "lambda." The
enzyme was an "exonuclease," so called because it functions by cutting
nucleotides off at the end of a DNA molecule. It cuts back only the 5′ end
of the nucleotide and as a result leaves a projecting single-stranded 3′ end

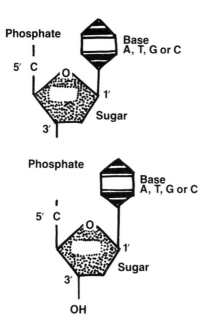

A nucleotide consists of a phosphate, a deoxyribose sugar, and one of four possible nitrogenous bases (A, C, G, or T). One of the latter attaches to the 1' carbon of the sugar. In DNA, adjacent nucleotides are joined by the phosphate between the 5' carbon atom of the sugar of one nucleotide and the 3' carbon atom of the sugar in the adjoining nucleotide. In DNA, one side of the double helix terminates in a 3' end while the other side, aligned in the opposite direction (antiparallel), terminates in a 5' end.

at each end of the linear DNA molecule. To these projecting 3' ends, a short series of identical nucleotides containing adenine were attached through the activity of another enzyme. Another batch of DNA was treated in a likewise manner, except that nucleotides containing thymine were added instead of adenine.

When these two samples of DNA were mixed, the complementary "tails" of A- and T-bearing nucleotides became joined by hydrogen bonding. This combined the once separate fragments into long, interconnected chains. DNA ligase was then added to form bonds between the sugar and phosphate groups. The two DNA strands were now one.

It was certainly intriguing that one could now cut up DNA into unpredictable heterogeneous fragments and randomly stitch them back together. However, for further insights into the organization of DNA and its genes—that is, the determination of precise nucleotide sequences— very specific nucleases would have to be found. The prevailing opinion was that such specific DNA-cutting capability did not exist in nature.

The only clue to the possibility that more specific nucleases might exist came from observations beginning as early as 1953 that when DNA molecules from *E. coli* were introduced into another slightly different form of *E. coli* they seldom functioned genetically. They were quickly broken down into smaller fragments. This apparently was part of a system that had evolved in bacteria to protect them against the entrance of foreign DNA. In addition to all of the other more obvious forms of competition in nature, there is a constant invisible struggle played out in the microscopic world, in this case between bacteria and bacteriophages. Darwin's natural selection is recreated here on a minute scale.

All organisms have developed some form of defense, including the simple expedient of growing rapidly. This will ensure that some will survive by the sheer weight of their numbers in spite of constant attack by predators. Bacteria are prime examples of this. In addition to their remarkable capacity to multiply rapidly, which in some species allows a population to double in size every 20 minutes, they produce enzymes which destroy incoming DNA from phage infection or from DNA picked up by other means.

These enzymes had been found by a series of investigators in a number of laboratories in the mid- and late-1960s. They named them "restriction endonucleases," or simply "restriction enzymes," since they cut up or "restricted" nucleic acids and were produced inside the cell. In 1970, Hamilton Smith of Johns Hopkins University followed up on his accidental discovery that the bacterium *Haemophilus influenzae* rapidly broke down phage DNA but would not harm its own genome. Study of cell-free extracts of this organism showed that the DNA degradation was caused by a restriction enzyme, which he and his colleagues isolated and named Hind II. This was the first in what would come to be known as a

```
5'  G   T   (C,T) ¦ (A,G)   A   C  3'
    |   |    |    ¦   |      |   |
3'  C   A   (G,A) ¦ (T,C)   T   G  5'
```

The enzyme Hind II cuts completely across the DNA double helix at a specific site.

series of Type II enzymes. Their use would revolutionize molecular biology.

Hind II was significantly different from the other restriction enzymes isolated earlier in that it was "site specific." That means that it had the very important characteristic of being able to recognize a specific nitrogenous base sequence and cut DNA apart at that site only.

Even more extraordinary was the EcoR I enzyme isolated soon afterward by Robert Yoshimori in Herbert Boyer's laboratory at the University of California School of Medicine at San Francisco. This enzyme induced breaks that were separated by several nucleotides. Each cut is always toward the 5' C end of a strand.

This enzyme cut the DNA only between G and A on the opposite sides of the helix. The helix broke apart at that point, leaving two ends with projecting complementary nucleotide sequences. These are known as "sticky ends" because the complementary sequences could easily stick together again by forming hydrogen bonds.

In November 1972, Janet Mertz and Ronald W. Davis of Stanford reported that viral DNA cleaved by EcoR I would rejoin first by hydrogen bonding and could be permanently held together by treatment with DNA ligase. The possibilities were staggering. Using this approach, could DNA from an organism be cut up and spliced to the DNA of another organism?

```
5'  G ¦ A   A   T   T   C  3'
    | ¦ |   |   |   |   |
3'  C   T   T   A   A ¦ G  5'
```

EcoR I cuts between G and A on opposite sides of the DNA double helix.

```
5′ G                    A A T T C ³′
   |      sticky end    sticky end    |
³′ C T T A A                        G  5′
```

The "sticky ends" are exposed nitrogenous bases.

In other words, could the natural barriers that prevent the exchange of genetic information between unrelated organisms be breached? These barriers have been built up over millions of years of evolution. Species are identified and determined by the genes that they carry. In organisms that breed sexually, species are literally defined by the ability of their members to breed with one another. This persistence of genetic uniqueness, rather than the chaos that would otherwise result, extends throughout the living world. Could this be overcome?

The answer was yes. The first step toward this was taken in 1973. A. C. Y. Chang and Stanley Cohen at the Stanford University School of Medicine and Herbert Boyer and Robert Helling at the University of California School of Medicine at San Francisco reported the joining of biologically functional DNA molecules from two different organisms. They called their composite molecule a DNA "chimera" because of its conceptual similarity to the mythological Chimera, a creature with the head of a lion, the body of a goat, and the tail of a serpent.

In this pioneering experiment, DNA fragments from *E. coli* were combined and inserted into other *E. coli* cells, whereupon the hybrid DNA functioned normally. Their chimeric DNA came to be known as recombinant DNA, or rDNA, and the process of cleavage, fusion, and replication of the chimera as "genetic engineering."

Note that in this first rDNA experiment, the DNA was not exchanged between species but from one *E. coli* to another. Using the procedures from their first success, the research group immediately went on to splice DNA from the dangerous bacterium *Staphylococcus* into *E. coli*. Given these successes, the question naturally arose—could animal genes also be introduced into bacteria and would they replicate and function there? They soon had the answer. Using DNA from a toad, they spliced a toad gene segment into *E. coli* DNA and put the newly made DNA into cells of the *E. coli* bacterium. Mythology had come to life. An animal–bacterial chimera had been created in the laboratory. The natural barriers between living kingdoms had been overcome.

Embodied in these three extraordinary experiments, simple in principle and introduced above in bare summary form, are the fundamental methods of the Human Genome Project. We must expand on these now in this context to promote a clear understanding of these procedures.

We have already explained the action of restriction enzymes. Since the properties of the original Hind II enzyme had been described and demonstrated by Huntington Smith in 1970, several hundred forms of these enzymes have been isolated and purified, each with its own specific sites of cleavage on the DNA molecule. These enzymes recognize a sequence of four to six nucleotides and most form a staggered cut on opposite sides of the double helix as in the case of EcoR I. Thus they leave sticky ends of unmatched nitrogenous bases. Now, 20 years later, one can simply peruse a molecular biology supply catalog, pick up a phone, and order any one of these enzymes.

Since the bases in the double helical DNA are complementary, the staggered pattern of cutting means, as we have pointed out, that half of the sticky ends are complementary to the other half. Therefore, theoretically, DNA from any other source—plant, animal, bacteria, and so on—cut with the same restriction enzyme will have these same complementary projecting sticky ends. When the two DNA samples are mixed under the proper conditions with DNA ligase added, the complementary bases will join by hydrogen bonding and the ligase will complete the repair of the helical backbones. In such a mixture, DNA from one source may fuse to DNA from the same source, or with foreign DNA.

The peculiar names of the restriction enzymes are derived in the following manner. The first three letters are taken from the Latin names of the bacterium from which they are isolated. The genus provides the first letter and the species the next two. *Haemophilus influenzae* becomes Hin and *Escherichia coli* becomes Eco. Sometimes a designation is included to indicate a specific form (strain) of a bacterium such as *Haemophilus* strain Rd in Hind or *E. coli* strain RY13, in EcoR. Often, more than one restriction enzyme is produced by one organism and each is numbered as it is isolated, as in Hind II or EcoR I.

Cutting and joining double-stranded molecules of DNA with enzymes was possible by 1972. But in order to do more than simply exist in a test tube as curiosities, these chimeras had to be placed within a DNA molecule that could replicate and function in a particular cell. The cell of choice has been the bacterial cell, for several reasons.

First, bacteria can be grown under controlled conditions, rapidly and in enormous numbers. Overnight, a few cells will multiply into literally billions. It is very important to understand that a bacterial cell ordinarily reproduces simply by copying itself. Assuming that no mutations occur in the cells, all the descendants of that one cell are identical. Such a population of cells originating from a single cell is termed a "clone" and the process of producing that clone is referred to as "cloning" the cell.

The DNA in a typical bacterial cell exists in two forms. One is the single bacterial chromosome which, unlike the chromosomes in our cells, is in the form of a circular molecule. The DNA of all other organisms can be likened to a long string. In bacteria, the ends of the string are joined, forming a circle. In addition to the DNA in the bacterial chromosome, DNA also occurs in bacteria in the form of plasmids. These, like the bacterial chromosome, are also circular DNA molecules, but much smaller. When the bacterial cell divides, the bacterial chromosome replicates and one chromosome is passed on to the new cell. Likewise, each of the plasmids replicate and half are delivered to the next generation. The plasmids are unique, independent, self-replicating DNA molecules which can exist only within the living bacterial cell.

Plasmid numbers average about 30 per cell and specific types of bacteria may have one per cell, others as many as several hundred. *E. coli* has 4.5 million nucleotide pairs in its chromosome while its plasmids may have only a few thousand. The human genome consists of 4 billion nucleotide pairs.

Plasmids can easily be isolated from bacteria by breaking open the cells with enzymes which break down the cell wall. The resulting mix is centrifuged. The heavier chromosomal DNA, termed "genomic" DNA, as well as cell fragments will go to the bottom. This leaves a relatively clean suspension of plasmids near the top of the centrifuge tube.

These tiny circles of DNA are actually not vital to the survival of the bacterium. The plasmids can be removed from a bacterial cell and the cell will function normally. However, some plasmids do contain genes which confer a marked advantage to the cell under certain conditions. For example, the fatal poison of "lockjaw" is a product of genes in plasmids of the tetanus bacterium. *E. coli* has plasmids that cause one form of the infamous "traveler's diarrhea."

Probably the most widely studied plasmid genes are the ones conferring resistance to specific antibiotics. Certain bacteria can produce enzymes coded for by plasmid genes that break down antibiotics such as penicillin, ampicillin, tetracycline, or chloramphenicol. In nature, this gives the bacteria a defense mechanism against naturally occurring antibiotics. In the tissues of an infected patient, bacteria with these plasmids may overcome the administration of therapeutic antibiotics. Such resistant infections have become a major medical problem.

This seemingly esoteric description of bacterial life contains another key element in our story. These bacterial plasmids are used as the DNA molecules into which other DNA fragments cut out by a restriction enzyme can be placed. Going back to our original principle, if we cut up any DNA with a restriction enzyme and cut plasmids with the same enzyme, mix the cut plasmids and the cut DNA in the presence of DNA ligase, plasmid–foreign DNA chimeras will be formed.

These chimeric plasmids, placed into receptive bacteria, will "live," that is, they will replicate and produce whatever gene products their constituent genes may code for. If the foreign DNA in the hybrid plasmid carries the proper code for protein x, then protein x will be produced. This amazing phenomenon demonstrates the remarkable unity of all living systems. Bacteria, ancient primitive organisms, have much the same cellular biochemistry as frogs, mice, trees, or humans. Given the almost universal code of genetic instructions, spelled out as nitrogenous base sequences, the bacterial cell, under the proper conditions, will assist in making a human protein as readily as a bacterial product.

Let us look once again at the very first recombinant DNA experiment done by Cohen and his co-workers in light of this more specific background. In so doing, we will explain the various steps necessary to carry out this deceptively simple experiment. Please keep in

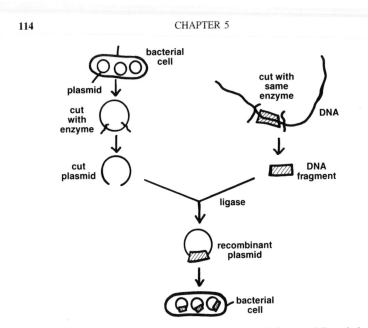

The DNA fragments will join to the cut plasmids by "sticky ends" made by the restriction enzymes. Placed back into bacteria, the new genes in the plasmids may be able to function as they would normally in the cells from which they come.

mind that the methods used in this now-classical experiment are indispensable tools in the mapping and sequencing of the human genome.

At Stanford University, Stanley Cohen had already isolated a wide variety of plasmids. One of them, pSC101, had the genetic information necessary to replicate in *E. coli* and to confer resistance to the antibiotic tetracycline.

One of the privileges of isolating plasmids is that one is allowed to name them. Plasmid pSC101 was the one hundred first (101) plasmid (p) isolated by Stanley Cohen (SC). Small though plasmids may be, their isolation and utilization may sometimes bring great rewards. Stanley Cohen shared the Nobel prize with Herbert Boyer and Paul Berg for their revolutionary recombinant DNA experiments.

Cohen and his co-workers had found that when they subjected the pSC101 plasmid to cleavage by EcoR I, it was cut in only one place, thus transforming the circular plasmid into a linear form. They reformed the plasmids into circles by joining the ends through the action of DNA ligase. They put them back into *E. coli* where the plasmids replicated as usual and thus were passed on to all the succeeding generations of those *E. coli*.

They were able to get the plasmids into the bacterial cells by the process of transformation. You will recall the original description by Fred Griffith of bacterial transformation back in 1928. In his experiment, DNA fragments from dead *Streptococcus* cells entered live cells and conferred on them the capacity to produce protective capsules. Such transformation occurs occasionally in nature in a few kinds of bacteria, among them *Streptococcus* of "strep-throat" fame.

In 1970, Morton Mandel and A. Higa at the University of Hawaii School of Medicine found that treatment of *E. coli* with calcium somehow enabled the bacteria to take up DNA extracted from viruses. In this receptive state the bacterial cells are referred to as "competent," which means that the DNA in the solution surrounding the cells will be absorbed through the wall and mingle with the cells' contents. *E. coli* is not naturally capable of transformation, but Cohen's group utilized this calcium technique and were able to introduce plasmids into *E. coli*. In this process, *E. coli* is first incubated so that it becomes a dense, rapidly growing population of healthy cells. The cells are spun down and resuspended in calcium chloride and then mixed with the DNA sample.

After being subjected to incubation at several different temperatures, the cells are spread out onto a solid growth medium suitable for *E. coli*, but that also contains tetracycline at a concentration that would ordinarily kill the cells. Those bacterial cells that have picked up one or more plasmids that confer antibiotic resistance will survive and multiply. Since bacteria multiply so rapidly, after overnight incubation individual clusters, each containing millions of cells, will be seen on the surface of the medium. These can be removed and put into a fresh growth medium to increase their numbers even further.

Essential to this procedure is that when bacteria are spread out on such a growth medium, each cell capable of growing will reproduce. As each cell resulting from successive reproductions heaps up upon its ancestors, they form a population of millions of cells which appear as a small spot on the solid medium surface.

This spot is a "colony" and a colony is a clone, a population of cells derived from one cell. All of the cells in this clone are identical, in theory at least, so that removing a colony and growing it in a flask or tube can supply one with a vast population of cells with the same genome.

Bacterial transformation actually occurs in only about one cell in a million during this laboratory procedure. However, using this technique, those few cells and their descendants in the form of colonies can be easily selected and readily propagated into as many cells as are needed for a particular purpose.

Stanley Cohen and his colleagues placed pSC101 plasmids into *E. coli* by transformation and the colonies of resistant cells were removed from tetracycline-containing solid medium. The next step was to see if a piece of foreign DNA could be inserted into the plasmids. EcoR I was used to cut open the DNA of another *E. coli* plasmid, this one carrying resistance to the antibiotic kanamycin. Then they mixed these plasmids with the pSC101 plasmids, also in linear form, and the sticky ends joined. The new plasmid hybrids were put into *E. coli*. Some of the bacteria survived on plates containing media with both tetracycline and kanamycin, a combination that ordinarily would have been lethal.

The plasmids that had resulted from their mixture were chimeras of pSC101 and a second DNA fragment from the other plasmid type that carried in its genes the information for producing resistance to kanamycin. This demonstrated, very importantly, that the pSC101 plasmid could serve as a carrier for introducing another DNA segment into *E. coli*. Many other such carriers have been developed since this first example. Such carriers are termed "vectors."

Was it possible that genes from another bacterial species could be combined with a carrier by such methods? Perhaps such bacterial DNA, being foreign to *E. coli*, would have genes which would not be able to function in such cells. Plasmid p1258, extracted from *Staphylococcus aureus*, conveyed resistance to yet another antibiotic, penicillin. This plasmid was cleaved with EcoR I and combined as above with pSC101. This new hybrid transformed *E. coli* into cells that were now tetracycline- and penicillin-resistant.

Finally, in this exciting series of experiments, the question was asked, "Could even animal cell genes be implanted in the bacteria, and would they function there?" Selecting a toad DNA fragment, they fused it to pSC101 and introduced the combination into *E. coli*. They then selected transformed colonies by their survival in a medium containing tetracycline. Since the new gene could not itself be conveniently selected out, the pSC101, with its tetracycline-resistant gene, was an effective vector for carrying it into the *E. coli* and also for selection.

The actual product produced by the activity of the new toad gene product was RNA, which ordinarily would be used to make a part of the toad cell's ribosome. In this case the *E. coli* reacted to the introduction of the newly created plasmid by obediently pumping out toad ribosomal RNA. The first animal–bacterial hybrid had been created.

The scientists involved and others who knew of their work immediately realized that the synthesis of novel gene combinations that had never before existed on the planet might have a potential for biological hazard. What if *E. coli* containing a dangerous gene were to escape from the lab and begin to infect human intestines? As researchers began to request samples of the plasmids from Cohen in order to pursue further recombinant studies, concerns arose as to the possibility of their producing bizarre combinations of DNA whose infectious properties and ecological effects could be unpredictable.

He sent the plasmids but asked for assurance that the recipients would neither introduce tumor viruses into bacteria nor create other dangerous bacteria that were not already in nature. In the summer of 1973, these growing concerns were broached at the annual Gordon Research Conference on Nucleic Acids held in New Hampshire.

Much concern focused on tumor-carrying viruses, which were then considered to be the only potential vectors for carrying rDNA into cells above the level of complexity of bacteria. The delegates voted to send a letter to the National Academy of Sciences (NAS), asking them to consider the problem of hazards and to recommend specific guidelines. Under the leadership of NIH researcher Maxine Singer and Deiter Söll of Yale University, a group of NAS scientists signed a letter that appeared simultaneously in the leading science journals *Nature*, *Science*, and *The*

Proceedings of the National Academy of Sciences. The letter was unprecedented in that it asked fellow scientists to declare a moratorium by deferring certain experiments, "until the potential of such recombinant DNA molecules have been better evaluated or until adequate methods are developed for preventing their spread."

One year later, another group, headed by Paul Berg of Stanford University, proposed that NIH devise guidelines for scientists who wished to continue research with potentially hazardous rDNA and also proposed that an international meeting be held early in 1975 to consider the matter more fully. The proposed meeting was held in February 1975 at the Asilomar Conference Center near Pacific Grove, California. It brought together 86 American biologists and 53 from 16 other countries. During the three and a half days of the conference the participants formulated guidelines that would allow most types of new genetic characteristics to be introduced into bacteria and viruses safely. Nonscientists from the fields of law and ethics also conferred.

The Asilomar recommendations included the use of physical containment barriers to protect lab workers and to prevent accidental escape of microorganisms into the environment. Also, they suggested that viruses be used that were specifically selected so that they could survive only in bacteria whose nutritional needs were so fastidious that they could live only under stringent laboratory conditions.

The day after the Asilomar Conference, the NIH Recombinant DNA Advisory Committee (RAC) convened and began work on what was to become a complex set of NIH guidelines. Their recommendations became official government regulations that took effect in July 1976. The basic theme of the guidelines was "to allow the promise of the methodology to be realized" while protecting against "what we and others view as potential hazards." In summary, the directives called for: (1) development of bacteria for use in these experiments that would die outside the laboratory environment; (2) a ban on five types of experiments deemed particularly dangerous; and (3) design of containment facilities for potentially hazardous experiments.

Volumes have been written about this era in molecular biology and it is not our purpose to recount the debate in detail. Basically, as experiments continued with no ill effects to either participants or the environment, there was a gradual relaxation of the guidelines. In fact, by 1981 most of the limits on rDNA using *E. coli* and yeast had been exempted from special lab controls. Often heated public debate accompanied the publication of the initial guidelines, and continued throughout the late 1970s. At times, entire communities debated the merits of banning such experiments within their boundaries.

As experimentation continued with no ill effects, scientific and public concern abated. Recombinant DNA research and related technologies became and continue to be the cutting edge of the biological sciences. As James Watson, regarding the guidelines initially banning the use of rDNA in the study of cancer genes, so laconically put it: "the[y] took force in July, 1976. They remained in effect until early in 1979. When they were relaxed, effective work on cancer viruses commenced."

For some, from radical activists to thoughtful scientists (not necessarily mutually exclusive categories), certain concerns remained. Those concerns included the adequacy of the environmental safeguards to protect against potentially hazardous effects which might result from the release of genetically engineered organisms. The original environmental impact guidelines were judged inadequate and in May 1984 were replaced by a very complex, and to some, cumbersome series of requirements, which had to be met before the deliberate release of such organisms. Weighed against the virtual impossibility of recalling bacteria once they have been released into the environment, it would seem that prudence in this complex area is the better part of impatience.

We have recounted the basic techniques developed in the early years of rDNA research. These included splicing of DNA fragments into bacterial plasmids followed by the insertion of those plasmids into bacteria. The transformed cells are selected by their new ability to resist antibiotics. All of these developments occurred in the late 1960s and early 1970s.

But, as we have asked before in other contexts, what of the gene? Could recombinant DNA techniques allow us finally to treat the gene as an individual molecular entity rather than as something buried somewhere in the chromosome? As a matter of fact, they could. So radical and powerful were these new tools that their use quickly became an international effort and remains so today.

As a result, scientists rapidly developed procedures for isolating and cloning individual genes. They were soon able to obtain large quantities of specific genes using a whole compendium of new approaches. This quickly led to the industrial and commercial application of genetic engineering known as "biotechnology."

The practice of biotechnology, although the name has a modern ring to it, is actually quite ancient. The term, in its general sense, refers to any technology that uses living organisms or parts of organisms to make or modify products to improve plants or animals or to develop microorganisms for specific uses. For centuries, humans have crossbred plants or animals to create hybrid forms with more desirable characteristics. The biotechnological practices of the fermenting of beer, wine, and cheese are ancient ones.

Modern biotechnology encompasses genetic engineering by making use of recombinant DNA. This involves direct manipulation of an organism's genetic material. Central to this effort is that genes direct the synthesis of gene products, the polypeptides of proteins. As a result, a gene inserted into a plasmid (or other DNA vector) and placed into bacteria will, under carefully controlled conditions, express itself by manufacturing that product within the bacterial cell. The applications are obvious. Already this technology has led, for example, to the production of proteins that dissolve blood clots, other proteins which may be used to control blood pressure or kidney function, hormones that reverse human dwarfism, and experimental vaccines. Given the correct gene, one can produce the polypeptide coded by that gene. As Francis Crick dryly put it, "Critics who previously had argued that few practical benefits had come from molecular biology were silenced by the realization that using these new techniques one could make money out of it."

In fact, the ability to obtain specific gene products has created a multibillion dollar industry. The resultant "brain-drain" of productive scientists from the academic ranks of genteel poverty to the status of entrepreneurs is a fascinating story. Certain aspects of that story, as they affect the Human Genome Project, will be treated in a later chapter.

          *   *   *

One bountiful harvest of the Human Genome Project will be a cornucopia of cloned human genes. Most of these will have never before been available and they will govern a multitude of human traits including a wide variety of diseases. Gene cloning procedures will allow these genes to be isolated and made available in large quantities. Many of the procedures used in gene cloning are central to genetic mapping and sequencing. Let us turn to how gene cloning is accomplished.

6

SEND IN THE CLONES

Chromosomes, seen through a microscope lens, offer little information to the viewer. The individual genes which make up the chromosomes are still invisible, just as a view of the earth from space reveals the continents, but none of the inhabitants. The precise location of the genes is thus hidden somewhere on those inert rods, scattered, stained, and fixed on the glass slide. We must leave behind the world of vision to find the genes.

At one level of analysis we might succeed in tracking them down to their neighborhood—a specific one of the 46 human chromosomes. This kind of basic "mapping" has already been done for almost 5000 genes. Searching even further, we might come upon the specific block in the neighborhood where they reside. The block will be crowded, but it will be, in biological terms, a chromosomal site that is accurate to within one million nitrogenous base pairs of its actual location on a particular chromosome. Relatively few genes as yet belong in this category.

Even more difficult to attain would be the ultimate goal of knowing the exact location of every gene—its home address. To accomplish that one would need to "sequence" the entire human genome, that is, to determine the nitrogenous base sequence of all of the nucleotides in human DNA. Yet that is precisely what the Human Genome Project proposes to do.

The results of such an analysis would be a string of 3 billion letters, A, T, G, or C, each representing the nitrogenous base of a nucleotide. A printout of simply the letters would fill 200 volumes the size of the Manhattan telephone book. Within that enormous list would be the sequence for every human gene as well as the sequence of great lengths of DNA with no currently known function.

Even the possession of such a sequence would be only the beginning. Knowing the sequence would not of itself tell us the location of all of our genes. Scientists would still want to know more. They want to find out not only the position but also the function of each gene and how that function is regulated and controlled.

For example, how do muscle cells, liver cells, or brain cells perform their individual and highly specialized functions using this same set of genes? Which genes become active or cease activity in these cells and how is that accomplished? Further, how does the myriad of cell types in the body unfold from only the fertilized human egg and its 46 chromosomes, half of which have been contributed by the mother and the other half by the father?

The simplest form of mapping is done by the more classical methods of analysis of the inheritance of visible characteristics in family histories. More detailed mapping and sequencing such as is being done in the Human Genome Project as well as related functional and developmental questions need and utilize the tools of molecular biology that we have introduced in the previous chapter.

In early 1990, the Department of Energy and the National Institutes of Health published the specific aims of the Human Genome Project with emphasis on the first five years extending from fiscal year 1991 to 1995. The publication spells out the scientific goals as well as the administrative framework proposed to assist in meeting them. Underlying all of the objectives is the absolute requirement for a supply of individual genes and groups of genes for detailed analysis.

Suppose that a geneticist working in 1970 had wanted to investigate the structure and function of the human genes governing the synthesis of hemoglobin, the oxygen-carrying molecule which gives color to our red blood cells. She might want to know the nitrogenous base sequence of those genes or perhaps determine what changes occur in the genes to cause the genetic disease thalassemia, in which one of the four polypeptides making up the hemoglobin molecule is not produced at all.

The question could not be answered unless enough of the gene could be provided to study it in detail—probably about a milligram, which amounts to about one forty-thousandths of an ounce. That sounds like a trifling amount but it becomes monumental when one considers purifying it from whole human DNA. The DNA involved in one hemoglobin gene is less than one part-per-million in the human genome. One would therefore need an unattainable amount of DNA as a starting material. If we assume that one could gather such a mass of human DNA, an even more difficult problem looms—how to separate the gene of interest from all the rest of the DNA?

Gene cloning now solves these problems. To clone a gene means simply to obtain a minute, pure sample of the gene and make lots more of it, as if one had a document and made many identical ones by photocopying it. The "photocopying" of genes is accomplished by first joining a few of the genes to vectors such as plasmids and inserting the vectors, now carrying the gene, into bacteria or other suitable cells.

We have introduced the basic principles of gene cloning already. In that process, so-called foreign DNA, the DNA we have removed from an organism, is inserted into the vector molecule, such as a plasmid, to create a DNA chimera. The building of such composites or artificial recombinant molecules has also been termed genetic engineering or "gene manipulation." This procedure has also been referred to as "molecular cloning" or "gene cloning" because a population of genetically identical bacteria, all containing the desired DNA, can be grown in great numbers, thereby copying the DNA as often as the cells divide.

What is very significant is that these chimeras within the bacterial cells may be able to copy not only themselves but actually produce a specific gene product in large amounts. This approach has already been utilized in the commercial production of human insulin, growth hormone, and the antiviral protein interferon. All of these can now be made by bacteria, because the human genes that regulate their synthesis have been isolated and cloned in bacteria. The bacterial cells, grown in vast numbers, obedient to the commands of their genes, now make a human gene product. Human gene products derived from genes isolated and cloned during the Human Genome Project will undoubtedly also be used for the benefit of humanity, particularly in the cure and prevention of disease.

However, our concern here is to examine the process of gene cloning enough to form a basis for a clear understanding of its essential use in realizing the goals of mapping and sequencing the human genome.

Let us first look at the arrangement of DNA within the chromosome as well as introduce the concept of how DNA function is regulated in the living cell. Living cells are of two fundamental types, procaryotic and eucaryotic. Procaryotic cells are bacteria while eucaryotic cells encompass all other cell types found in living organisms.

A major distinction between these two categories is that the bacteria do not have a membrane separating the chromosome DNA from the rest of the cell contents as do the eucaryotes. In other words, bacterial cells do not have a nucleus. Also, bacteria have about one-thousandth as much DNA as the typical eucaryotic cell. DNA in eucaryotic cells is a long, thin double helix within the cell nucleus. In contrast, bacterial DNA is simply concentrated in a central region of the cell.

This bacterial genome is a single chromosome, a double helix in the form of a ring like a DNA snake with its tail in its mouth. It has very little protein associated with it, in contrast to the human genome in which protein makes up a significant part of the chromosome. Bacterial cells also may house smaller DNA rings, the plasmids, which are independent from the chromosome in replication and function. The basic pattern of replication of DNA and the translation of genetic messages into proteins are in many respects the same for both pro- and eucaryotes but important differences remain.

The understanding of these differences is particularly significant in gene cloning. Remember, in this procedure, we are often placing eucaryotic genes into a bacterial cell. The survival and function of those introduced genes depends upon the control of certain parameters which reflect these pro/eucaryotic differences.

When human chromosomes are observed through the microscope they look like bent, dark rods. Typically, chromosomes are examined after they have been preserved in alcohol, stained with dyes, and spread out on a glass microscope slide. Moreover, in order to be seen clearly these chromosomes must be caught in the act of cell division (mitosis). Only in this brief period in the life of the cell do the chromosomes, normally elongated and nearly invisible in the nondividing cell, coil and condense into typical blunt shapes.

Each of the 23 chromosome pairs assumes a unique shape in this process, so that one can prepare a "karyotype" of human chromosomes. This evolves from photographing the chromosomes from a dividing cell and arranging them in 23 separate pairs in order of their size and shape. This is a valuable aid in the diagnosis of such disorders as a missing or partial chromosome. Obviously, the presence of two X chromosomes or an X and a Y determines the individual as a female or male and leads to a routine method for a prenatal diagnosis of sex.

Human chromosomes are about 60% protein and 40% DNA. Some RNA is also present because of the occurrence of messenger RNA synthesis. As noted earlier, the DNA of the chromosome exists as one long, unbroken double-helix strand. A typical human chromosome contains about 140 million nucleotide pairs. Stretched out, the chromosome would be about 2 inches long. Obviously an enormous amount of coiling is necessary to fit 46 chromosomes into the cell's small nucleus.

If we could gently uncoil a human chromosome, we would find that it would resemble beads on a string, with the string being the DNA and the beads the proteins. Every 200 nucleotides the DNA helix is wrapped around a complex of "histones" which are small polypeptides. These proteins are positively charged and the DNA is negatively charged and is thus strongly attracted to the protein cluster. Further coiling of the DNA occurs as the string of DNA and histones wraps up into "supercoils."

This condensation is necessary so that the chromosome can pass intact from one cell to the next as cell division proceeds. The actual doubling of the DNA molecule occurs when it is in the partly uncoiled state. As the chromosomes condense to small thick rods by coiling, they have already replicated and appear as joined pairs, each chromosome still bound to the new replicate at a region termed the centromere.

In terms of function, we need to make a few distinctions beyond the generality that the chromosome is a DNA molecule made of genes that directs the synthesis of polypeptides. To add to the complexity of analysis of human and other eucaryotic DNA, approximately 10 to 25% of the total DNA is made up of short sequences typically five to ten nucleotides long that are repeated in tandem thousands of times. In the chromosomes these tandem repeats are located at the centromeres where the two chromosomes remain attached after replication until they separate as the

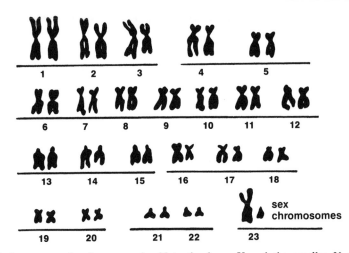

A karyotype of a human male. Note the large X and the smaller Y sex chromosomes. Each chromosome appears double because the karyotype is made after the chromosomes have replicated before mitosis but have not yet separated.

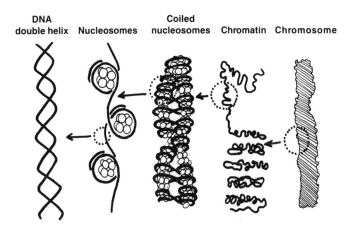

A chromosome, in the stage when it can be seen with a microscope, is a tightly coiled DNA molecule which is itself coiled around clusters of protein molecules.

cell divides. Apparently, this area of DNA serves a structural rather than a genetic role in the cell and somehow operates during replication and separation.

We have already described how, after the initial concerns about the safety of recombinant DNA had abated and researchers began to use safe vectors to study the structure of chromosomes in earnest in 1977, a surprising discovery was made. Patterns of restriction-enzyme-produced fragments of eucaryotic chromosomal DNA revealed that there were regions scattered within the genes that were not part of the gene at all. They were sequences of nucleotides which appeared to have no function whatsoever. In contrast, a bacterial gene is simple. It is uninterrupted so that the code of the gene can be directly interpreted from the amino acid sequence of the polypeptide whose synthesis it directs.

No one had assumed eucaryotes would be any different, but they are. Eucaryotic genes are often arranged in pieces, separated by so-called "nonsense" codes. Walter Gilbert of Harvard University termed these intervening sequences "introns" and the sequence of the actual gene codes as "exons." Try adding a few dozen extra digits at random here and there within your telephone number. Your number would be the exons, and all the rest would be the introns.

Some genes have no introns; others have many. No one knows for sure why we have introns. Curiously, for reasons yet unknown, the human gene in which the most introns have been found to date is the gene whose failure causes Duchenne muscular dystrophy. It has at least 60 to 100 introns. When, as the RNA prepares to carry the gene code information out of the nucleus, messenger RNA is synthesized along the length of an entire gene, the introns form parts of the RNA as well. Then the introns are enzymatically cut out in a process known as RNA splicing. This leaves the messenger RNA with a reflection of the code of the gene and not the introns.

This phenomenon points out two problems associated with gene cloning. One is that it is not possible to infer from the amino acid sequence in a protein the exact nitrogenous base sequence in that segment of the chromosome from which it was coded. The introns will not be reflected in the amino acid sequence since they have been cut out of the message. Also, one must manipulate the experimental conditions during cloning so that the bacteria are able to overcome the presence of introns in the DNA, since bacteria do not have introns in their chromosomes.

Moreover, how do cells, both procaryotic and eucaryotic, see to it that certain genes are active and others are not? Cells must be able, at least, to "repress" genes, otherwise chaos would result. All of our cells, except the sperm and eggs, have a complete set of our genes. Eye cells have genes for kidney function, while heart cells have genes for hair color. Cells have somehow evolved mechanisms to repress the genes coding for enzymes that are not needed at any one time and to activate the genes when they are needed. The elucidation of these systems remains a major area of research in molecular biology. Quite frankly, scientists as yet know very little about how such complex systems operate. However, we can relate a few known generalities relevant to this question.

François Jacob and Jacques Monod of the Institut Pasteur in Paris were the pioneers in the 1950s and 1960s in the study of these questions with their masterful Nobel-winning analysis of how *E. coli* makes enzymes that break apart lactose (milk sugar) molecules. The products of this breakdown are used as a source of nutrition by the bacteria. Among other conclusions, they found that in order for messenger RNA to be synthesized at the gene, the enzyme RNA polymerase must bind to the DNA near the beginning of the gene at a region called the promoter. The enzyme then quickly begins to put together the messenger RNA needed to synthesize the enzymes required to break down the lactose.

The eucaryotic cell has requirements for gene control of even greater complexity. Not only must the genes be turned on or off to operate basic cell functions but these systems also must respond to signals from the cells' surroundings. This is especially important in cells that are differentiating into various cell types. A fertilized human egg becomes a baby, a creature made up of trillions of cells of many kinds. Somehow, each developmental stage triggers the gene expression needed for the next stage.

In human cells with their 100,000 genes, at any one time only about 1% of the genome is actually expressing itself. The other 99% is turned off by systems only now being uncovered through molecular biological techniques. For our purposes, let us simply generalize that regulatory systems similar to those in bacteria are involved—but there are many additional complexities. Again, most questions surrounding this complicated area remain unanswered.

There are differences between the promoter sequences in bacteria and those in eucaryotes, which latter group includes humans. The promoters for messenger RNA synthesis in the human genome are not necessarily recognized by bacteria. In order to obtain expression of a human DNA sequence inserted into *E. coli*, for example, it may be necessary to position the human gene next to a bacterial promoter.

In addition, to achieve expression of eucaryotic DNA in bacteria, it is necessary to add a site on the recombinant DNA molecule allowing it to bind to the bacterial ribosomes. This binding site is not normally present in eucaryotic DNA. In summary, it is not sufficient to include only the human DNA genes in gene cloning, at least if one proposes to use them to express themselves in polypeptide synthesis. A mosaic of accessories must be engineered to accompany the gene in question, which makes genetic engineering more complicated than it might seem at first.

If the scientist is interested only in obtaining large quantities of the gene rather than making a gene product, it is sufficient if the gene is simply copied in the vector.

Now, having seen some of the complexities that need to be dealt with, let's turn to some practical considerations in cloning human genes. Any DNA cloning procedure has four basic parts: (1) a method for making DNA fragments, (2) joining of these "foreign" DNA fragments to the vector, (3) a means of introducing this recombinant into a host cell where it can replicate, and (4) a method for "screening" or selecting a clone of cells that have acquired the recombinant. We followed those steps in our recounting of the very first recombinant DNA experiments of the early 1970s.

Suppose we want to follow those basic steps in order to clone human genes. Because of the size and complexity of the human genome, more sophisticated methods and strategies have been and continue to be developed for such a task.

There are two basic approaches to cloning a specific gene. They have to do with the starting material. The first approach involves cloning all the DNA fragments from a DNA sample cut into pieces by restriction enzymes. Then the pieces are put into bacteria, cloned, and the bacteria with the various DNA fragments are selected out, usually by their antibiotic resistance. Then the clones with the actual gene one is interested in are selected by a means which we will explain shortly. This practice of cloning all the random DNA fragments of a DNA sample is called "shotgunning."

For example, we might digest total human DNA with a restriction enzyme, insert each fragment or small groups of fragments into a suitable vector, clone, and then attempt to isolate the clones containing a specific gene. This is roughly equivalent to passing the Sunday *New York Times* through a shredder, making a few million photocopies of each piece, mixing everything together, and looking for the pieces with the Mets' score.

Let us assume that the DNA fragments resulting from enzyme digestion were, on the average, about 1000 to 2000 base pairs long, or, to use the conventional term, 1 to 2 "kilobases" (kb) long. Since human DNA contains approximately 3 billion base pairs, the concentration of any specific DNA fragment would be less than one in a million, making this a cumbersome approach to the problem. There would be a limited number of pieces of sports pages in our shredded pile and they would be far outnumbered by an overwhelming mass of extraneous fragments.

This problem can at least be somewhat alleviated by cloning random fragments of a larger size, for example, about 20 kb. This fragmentation could be done by mechanically breaking up the DNA, but more commonly the DNA is treated with either one or sometimes a mixture of two restriction enzymes. This is allowed to proceed only to a state of partial digestion, producing fragments that are in the range of 10 to 30 kb. These can be treated to separate out the fragments that are about 20 kb in size and these then can be inserted into a simple vector. It has been calculated that about one million clones would be needed to ensure a 90–95% chance that every one of the 20-kb fragments would be included. Let's adjust the blades on our shredder so that the pieces produced are bigger. At least we'll have fewer to search through.

Regardless of the exact method used, a collection of random DNA fragments that are put into a vector and cloned is referred to as a "gene library" or sometimes a "genomic library" or "gene bank." This library is a complete set of clones containing the totality of the genome. Our exposure to clones thus far has been clones in the form of transformed bacterial colonies. We'll put all identical photocopied pieces of our newspaper into, let's say, a million folders. The gene library is a valuable resource of human DNA fragments for mapping and sequencing. Once established, it serves as a means of maintaining a consistent supply of DNA for research.

The second approach to cloning a specific gene is in marked contrast to the use of genomic clones. It involves creating much more specific DNA segments, termed complementary DNA or cDNA. It takes advantage of the fact that, because of the way proteins are made, the nitrogenous base sequence of messenger RNA is a direct complement to the sequence of the actual gene.

Because of that fact, cDNA can be synthesized by using its mRNA. The "Central Dogma" that DNA makes RNA makes protein experienced a sudden transition from a universal statement to a generality in 1970. In that year, Howard Temin and David Baltimore independently discovered the enzyme "reverse transcriptase." It was found in certain types of viruses, the "retroviruses," that contain RNA rather than DNA. The retroviruses include in their number such important pathogens as certain hepatitis and leukemia viruses, as well as the infamous causative agent of AIDS known officially as the human immunodeficiency virus (HIV).

In this form of viral attack, RNA, and not DNA, enters the eucaryotic cell. The reverse transcriptase enzyme uses the RNA of the virus as a template to form a complementary single strand of DNA, literally making one side of the ordinarily two-sided double helix. The latter then serves as a template for the formation of a second strand complementary to it, thereby forming a double-stranded DNA. This DNA then actually enters the chromosomal DNA of the host cell where it is replicated during cell divisions. Later (in the case of AIDS, sometimes many years later), this DNA becomes active and directs the synthesis of new, infectious retroviral particles which leave the cell and enter other cells.

In carrying out the mRNA to cDNA synthesis in the laboratory, it makes sense to obtain the mRNA from cells in which the gene that one is trying to clone is highly active. For example, cells in the human pancreas contain relatively high concentrations of mRNA that help make insulin, and the cells that mature into red blood cells are rich in mRNA because they are carrying the message for the gene in charge of making hemoglobin. As a result, isolation of mRNA from such cells provides an enriched sample of specific mRNA. Almost pure hemoglobin mRNA can readily be prepared from immature red blood cells. With reverse transcriptase, cDNA can be prepared and used as the DNA source for further cloning.

Now that we have a source of DNA for cloning, whether it be large fragments or much more specific cDNA molecules, a suitable cloning vector for our human DNA must be selected. We have already described the use of plasmids such as pSC101 in the early days of the revolutionary technique of recombinant DNA. After their initial successes, Boyer and his colleagues developed a set of very popular vectors known as the pBR series. In creating plasmids for use as cloning vectors, several characteristics are desirable.

One is the ability of the plasmid to function as a "high copy plasmid," that is, the capacity to copy itself repeatedly in the cell, sometimes as many as 1000 times. This, of course, greatly increases the final yield of genes carried by those plasmids. In addition, the plasmid should have a system to demonstrate the presence of foreign DNA inserts. You will recall that the first such marker was resistance to an antibiotic. A variety of antibiotic-resistant factors have been engineered into plasmid vectors. One of these plasmids, pBR322, has been widely used. It has a high copy number and has two genes for antibiotic resistance—both to tetracycline and to ampicillin.

Modifications of pBR322 were used by Boyer's group in 1977 in their synthesis of the human gene which makes human growth regulating hormone. The gene was cloned and the hormone is now available to the medical community. In August 1990 researchers reported that, in a clinical trial, treatment of elderly persons with the growth regulating hormone dramatically reversed several characteristics of aging including skin and muscle tone.

While commonly used to carry relatively small DNA fragments, plasmids are limited by the size of the DNA that they can carry. Plasmids typically can carry DNA sequences of up to 12 kb. Larger DNA segments can be carried by the DNA molecule derived from the well-known lambda phage. This has been engineered to be particularly useful for human genome analysis.

Such vectors have been named by their creator Fred Blattner "Charon" phages. Charon, another mythological figure, is the boatman on the river Styx. Just as Charon ferries souls to the underworld, the Charon phage carries DNA to the bacterial cells. The most common use for the Charon phages is in the construction of genomic libraries. The phages have been cleverly engineered to accept only DNA between 12 and 20 kb. That assures that clones with insignificant amounts of DNA do not clutter up the library. Even at that, at 12 to 20 kb per clone one needs about a million clones for a complete library.

Other vectors have been developed for specialized purposes, such as "cosmid" vectors for carrying DNA fragments of up to 40–50 kb. Recently, a relatively new form of vector has been gaining increasing use in human genome analysis. It is the "YAC," or yeast artifical chromosome, developed in 1987 by David T. Burke, George F. Carle, and Maynard V. Olson at the Washington University School of Medicine. A major advantage in cloning genes in yeast is the ability to clone large pieces of DNA. Many human DNA sequences of interest are quite large. For example, the gene for the blood clotting factor VIII covers about 190 kb or about 0.1% of the human X chromosome and the Duchenne muscular dystrophy gene covers more than 1 million bases.

The YAC is DNA ingeniously engineered by assembling the essential functional parts of a natural yeast chromosome. A fragment of human DNA is spliced into this and the chromosome is inserted into a yeast cell where the YAC is reproduced during cell division. The result is a DNA clone within yeast cells rather than bacterial cells. So widespread has the use of yeast become in genetic analysis that James Watson, in his textbook of molecular genetics *The Molecular Biology of the Gene*, calls yeast ". . . the *E. coli* of eucaryotic cells."

The 1990 Department of Energy/National Institutes of Health five-year plan includes a major effort to improve the available YAC vectors and the YAC cloning procedures, particularly as regards increasing the size of the DNA fragments that can be cloned as well as further improvements in methods to later separate them from the yeast.

Regardless of the specific method selected in the preparation of gene libraries or in the cloning of cells containing specific gene sequences of interest, scientists are left with a final analytical problem. A convenient method is needed for separating and analyzing the many thousands of fragments in the gene library, deciding which transformed cells actually contain the desired gene, and separating that gene from all of the other DNA in the sample. Which folders contain the Mets' score? There are one million and they all look alike.

A method is now available. It is "gel electrophoresis," a method which can identify DNA in concentrations as low as 10 nanograms (one hundred millionth of a gram). This has become an extraordinarily valuable tool of molecular biology and is indispensable in almost every aspect of genetic manipulation.

We have already recounted how, in 1949, a research team led by Linus Pauling demonstrated that normal and sickle-cell hemoglobin migrated at different rates in a solution exposed to an electric field. In this way they deciphered the molecular abnormality causing sickle-cell anemia, the most common genetic disease among blacks. Forty years later, gel electrophoresis, a highly refined modification of Pauling's technique, pinpointed the differences in DNA sequences between healthy volunteers and people suffering from cystic fibrosis, the most common genetic disease among whites.

In electrophoresis, molecules are placed in an electric field and allowed to migrate toward the positive or negative poles. The molecules separate because they move at different rates depending on their differences in charge and size. In gel electrophoresis, the mixture to be separated is placed into a small depression molded into the end of a thin sheet of a gel bathed in a solution. The gel is made of either agarose or polyacrylamide.

Agarose is a natural complex sugar extracted from certain species of red seaweed. When dissolved and then poured to form a thin layer on a glass plate, it solidifies into a gel with relatively large pores. Agarose gel electrophoresis (AGE) is convenient for separating DNA fragments ranging in size from a few hundred to about 20 kb.

Polyacrylamide is preferred for smaller DNA fragments ranging from 1000 down to 6 base pairs. It is a synthetic gel made by mixing acrylamide with a chemical agent that creates a gel with a uniform pore size. The small pore size possible in these gels is critical in DNA sequence analysis, making polyacrylamide gel electrophoresis (PAGE) essential to DNA sequencing studies.

Both agarose and polyacrylamide gels are porous substances through which molecules slowly move in response to an applied electric field. Pores in the gel limit the movement of large molecules while smaller molecules migrate more freely and therefore travel farther. This gradually results in a separation of molecules based on a combination of their size and electrical charge.

DNA fragments, because of their phosphate groups, carry negative charges and so migrate toward the positive pole. The small fragments move the farthest and the largest the least. After this separation, which typically takes several hours, the DNA fragments have been spread out along a narrow path or "lane" in the gel. In order to see the ordinarily invisible DNA, the gel can be treated with a dye that binds to DNA and fluoresces in ultraviolet light. The DNA spots scattered along the gel lane can be seen by placing the gel on an ultraviolet light box. Each beautiful glowing spot is a mass of DNA fragments of a specific size, with the largest fragments the ones having moved the least and the smallest those that have raced to the farthest region of the lane.

A control mixture of known DNA fragment sizes is run simultaneously in a separate lane. One can then readily calculate the size of the DNA in each spot by comparing them to the distribution of the fragments of known molecular size. Our analogy stumbles a bit as we cannot put our folders onto a gel. Instead, lets have someone separate them into piles. Each pile will contain folders that contain all the pieces of pages from just one of the various sections of the paper. Now, one of the piles will include all of the sports pages. (Yes, this would be a horrendous task. Electrophoresis is much easier.)

Recent innovations have allowed the electrophoresis of very large DNA molecules, which in the past have been impossible to separate on conventional gels. In agarose gel electrophoresis, DNA larger than 50 kb tends to run together at the same speed. In 1984, in an effort to find a method to separate yeast chromosomes, Charles Cantor and D. C.

Schwartz of Columbia University invented "pulsed-field gel electro-phoresis" (PFGE).

In this modification the strength and direction of the applied electric field is varied rapidly with time. The larger the DNA fragment, the longer it takes to realign itself to a new migration direction. This results in the eventual separation of very large pieces of DNA. PFGE has become the universal means of separating DNA fragments of up to 10 million base pairs. PFGE and its several variations were instrumental in 1989 in allowing the mapping of the cystic fibrosis gene and then in 1990 the gene causing Wilms' tumor, a kidney tumor occurring in children. Further refinement of PAGE involving computer-assisted control is another goal of the DOE/NIH five-year plan.

In summary, gel electrophoresis in its various forms is used to separate DNA fragments. Just as coins dumped into a bank's coin sorter drop through holes of a particular diameter and form neat stacks of pennies, nickels, dimes, and quarters, the various categories of DNA fragment sizes end up in neat piles along the length of the gel lane.

One is still left with the problem of locating a specific gene once it has been cloned. How can one reach into the gel and extract specific genes, distinguishing them from all other DNA present? Which pile of folders contains our long-awaited score? Whoever separated them into piles is sworn to secrecy.

The answer lies in the use of a "probe," often in conjunction with gel electrophoresis. Remember, we have taken DNA fragments randomly, or perhaps more specifically in the case of cDNA, and inserted them into a vector. The vector has been put into bacteria which have cloned the DNA fragments. By selection methods such as antibiotic resistance those clones of bacterial cells containing newly introduced DNA are selected.

If random DNA fragments have been put in the vectors, only some of the clones will contain the gene that we want. We must probe for the gene as a magnet might probe out a piece of iron among the rubble.

A probe (the magnet) is a segment of DNA or RNA which is known to be complementary, at least in part, to the gene (the iron) which we wish to isolate. The use of such a probe is called nucleic acid "hybridization." This is based on the now-familiar fact that chromosomal DNA occurs as a double-stranded molecule—remember the ladder analogy. If the two strands are separated by breaking the hydrogen bonds that hold the nitrogenous bases together, any strand of DNA or RNA complementary nucleotides can, under the appropriate conditions, attach to those exposed nitrogenous bases and form a "hybrid" double-stranded DNA or DNA/RNA hybrid.

The probe can be labeled, for example, by being supplied with radioactive molecules during its synthesis. The presence of hybridization can then be detected by detecting the radiation. The use of nucleic acid hybridization is absolutely central to the practice of molecular genetics, including mapping and sequencing.

Let us look at several common variations on the use of probes. First we will assume that we have colonies of transformed bacteria growing on a solid culture medium. A small sample of cells from each colony is transferred and spotted onto another plate in a gridlike arrangement. Overnight, the transferred cells grow into colonies. An absorbent pad is placed over the surface of the medium where the bacterial colonies are growing and then carefully removed.

Some bacterial cells adhere to the pad, forming the same grid pattern on the pad that they had on the medium. The pad is then treated with a dilute solution which will denature the DNA, that is, open it up, separating the two sides of the double helix. The DNA is bound firmly to the pad by a heat treatment. Finally, the pad is placed into a dish containing the radioactive probe. The probe will cling only to complementary base sequences. The iron fragments now cling to the magnet.

The pad is rinsed thoroughly to remove any unattached probe and in the darkroom an X-ray film is placed next to the pad. Wherever radioactively labeled probe is bound to the pad it exposes the film, producing a dark spot. These spots correspond to the position of the colonies containing the gene of interest. One can go back to the original colony, remove it, and culture it to produce as much of the gene as one wishes.

Another extraordinarily valuable technique for probing for genes in genetic mapping studies was developed by E. M. Southern in 1975. This procedure, now known as "Southern blotting," begins with the separation of restriction-enzyme-digested DNA by gel electrophoresis. As we have shown, the DNA pieces spread out along the gel lane according to their size. The location of a particular gene in one of the resulting DNA bands follows in principle the same protocol as above.

That is, the absorbent pad is laid in this case onto the gel and covered with dry filter paper. This causes some of the DNA fragments to be leached out of the gel onto the filter. Treatment of the filter with the appropriate probe will locate the particular spot on the lane in which the gene is located. The spot can literally be cut out of the gel and the DNA extracted from the gel. The cloned genes are now in a test tube, at our disposal.

How can we "probe" for our piece of newspaper? We'll just have to use poetic license and assume that we have conjured up a method to "label" the Mets' score by inserting iron filings into the ink used to print it. By applying a magnet as a probe we can easily pull out all the pieces on which the score appears. They lost, 9 to 0.

Gene cloning, as we have just described it, even for those quite familiar with it, is a complex, time-consuming, and labor-intensive technique. It often means growing bacteria, the use of vectors, selection of colonies, radioactive probes, and so forth. Of course, if you consider the importance of the extraordinary feat that gene cloning accomplishes, you can see why such efforts are gladly undertaken.

In the mid-1980s, a revolutionary method for accomplishing the same feat became available. It is, in fact, considered to be the most dramatic development to come out of molecular biology in that decade. It is the "polymerase chain reaction," or PCR.

With PCR one needs only a minute amount of DNA and unlimited copies of the DNA can be made—by machine. PCR is a method whose component parts had long been known to molecular biologists but whose brilliant synthesis occurred late one Friday night in April 1983 as a young man drove along a moonlit road into northern California's redwood country. In a flash of insight reminiscent of Watson's experience in the last stages of his DNA model building, Kary Mullis hit upon a method in which minuscule amounts of DNA could be quickly amplified into large quantities—in a few hours.

The method came into widespread use in 1988 and already promises to replace traditional gene cloning as the method of choice for gene sequencing. PCR is now absolutely essential to the Human Genome Project. Let's look briefly at how it works.

The polymerase chain reaction can be utilized to copy a solitary molecule of DNA many millions of times in a few hours. The procedure is simple—a few reagents, some heat, and some DNA to copy. The DNA may come from anywhere: a plasmid, a cell, or perhaps even a single human hair or a drop of blood. It can be done in a test tube or (given the budget) in an automatic analyzer the size of a desktop computer.

In addition to the kinds of probes which we have just described there is another very useful kind of probe called an "oligonucleotide," or to the in crowd, an "oligo." It is simply a short chain of nucleotides of known nitrogenous base sequence which can be made to order in the laboratory. It will attach to any single-stranded DNA to which it is complementary. Again, picture the DNA double helix as a ladder. Cut the rungs in half and the two sidepieces of the ladder with their projecting rung segments separate from each other. Each ladder half now represents a single-stranded DNA as opposed to the double-stranded intact ladder. The projecting rung halves are the nitrogenous bases, now exposed and each available for attachment to a complementary base.

In 1979, the CETUS Corporation in Emeryville, California hired Kary Mullis to make oligo probes, the sale of which was becoming a thriving business. After earning his Ph.D. in biochemistry from the University of California at Berkeley, Mullis had done postdoctoral work at the University of Kansas Medical School and the University of

oligonucleotide
3′ G C G A 5′
   | | | |
5′ T C G A C G C T 3′
single stranded DNA

An oligonucleotide can attach to the complementary bases on single-stranded DNA. This single strand is made by splitting apart the double helix, easily accomplished by heating.

California at San Francisco. Oligo synthesis had advanced from manual synthesis to rapid automated synthesis. The tedium of loading and unloading probe synthesizers gave Mullis time to "tinker."

Mullis decided to try to work out a scheme in his spare time for easily determining the identity of a nucleotide at any given position on a DNA molecule. From his experience in trying to determine DNA sequences, a most laborious task at that time, he knew of two methods that might work together in a single experiment.

In 1955, Arthur Kornberg and his colleagues at Stanford University had isolated the naturally occurring cellular enzyme DNA polymerase. The enzyme has several functions in the cell, including replication of DNA, as well as DNA "repair." Such repair is necessary on a regular basis because DNA is subject to damage as it replicates and functions within the nucleus. It is estimated that up to 5000 purine bases (A or G) are lost each day from the DNA in every human cell because heat breaks the bonds linking them to deoxyribose. Enzymes remove the damaged areas and DNA polymerase helps to synthesize new nucleotides whose nitrogenous bases are complementary to those on the strand opposite the damaged portion.

It so happens that DNA polymerase can also lengthen a short oligo strand, in this case called a "primer," by attaching a nucleotide to its 3' end. The only requirement is that the primer has to be bound to a complementary single-stranded DNA. That is certainly simple enough to do. The portion of the DNA "ladder" with the primer now attached is an intact ladder segment, that is, double-stranded DNA. As each oligo is added the "ladder repair" continues.

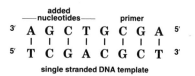

Starting at the oligonucleotide primer, nucleotides are added in a sequence that is determined by the sequence of the exposed nitrogenous bases on the single-stranded DNA.

Also, in order for this addition of nucleotides, a supply of nucleotides as building blocks is obviously required. These can easily be supplied. Such nucleotides are called deoxyribonucleotide phosphates (dNTPs) and, since there are four possible nitrogenous bases, there are four possible dNTP forms, each one containing a different base. This includes dATP, dGTP, dCTP, or dTTP containing respectively adenine, guanine, cytosine, or thymine.

Now, instead of supplying the reaction mixture with dNTPs, one can add instead a slightly different form of nucleotide called a dideoxy-ribonucleotide phosphate (ddNTP). There are four forms of these as well, ddATP, ddGTP, ddCTP, and ddTTP. These are similar to dNTPs except for the fact that they will not allow the addition of any further nucleotides to the chain. So, once a ddNTP is added to the primer, no more can be added. Therefore, once a ddNTP is added on next to the primer, no further addition of nucleotides can occur. No more rungs of the ladder can be rejoined.

Based on these reactions, already long familiar to molecular biologists, Mullis reasoned that if he could determine which of the four ddNTPs had been added to the primer, he would then know the identity of the corresponding nitrogenous base in the template strand.

As Kary Mullis drove north on that evening in April, anticipating a restful weekend in his cabin three hours away in the hills, he thought that his proposed technique seemed to be a reasonably simple and straightforward procedure. He would separate a DNA fragment into single strands by heating it. Then he would bind an oligo primer to a complementary sequence on one of the strands and place portions of the mixture into four different test tubes. Each tube would contain all four types of ddNTP but

The ddTTP blocks the addition of any more nucleotides onto the exposed single strand of DNA.

in each tube a different one of the four forms of the ddNTP would be radioactively labeled.

Next, by adding DNA polymerase the primer would be extended by the addition of one ddNTP and no more nucleotides could be added. Gel electrophoresis could be used to analyze the contents of each tube to see which had added a radioactive ddNTP. If it was one containing A, then it had attached to a T on the DNA strand, if it contained G, then it had attached to a C, and so on.

Simple enough. But to be sure of his results should he perhaps add two oligos, one on each end of the two separated DNA single strands? He might as well use both sides of the double helix to make sure of his answer.

Then came the "eureka" moment. He was suddenly struck by the realization that if he simply attached the primers some distance apart on opposite sides of the helix, added a supply of all four kinds of dNTPs, then the double strand made by the step-by-step extension of the primers would have the same base sequence as the original DNA. This reaction would double the number of DNA strands in the sample. It would clone that part of the DNA!

Moreover, after a few rounds of extending the primers, separating the double strand produced, adding new primers and extending them, more and more cloned DNA would be made. Large segments of DNA could be synthesized merely by designing primers that bound far apart on the opposite DNA strands of the double helix, rather than one base apart. An entire intact ladder could be made by starting the ladder repair at either end on opposite ladder halves. DNA could be cloned in a test tube.

Back at CETUS on Monday morning, Mullis began to define the optimum conditions for the reaction. It worked just as theory indicated that it would. DNA, for all practical purposes, could be "photocopied." When the procedure was published and the details became known, the universal response of molecular biologists was "Why didn't I think of that?"

PCR is now automated, enabling the copying of DNA segments up to several thousand bases in length. Prior to 1988, PCR was a rather tedious procedure due to the fact that the DNA polymerase was destroyed at each heating step, necessitating the addition of new polymerase. In

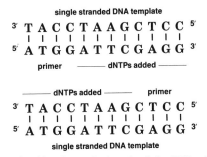

single stranded DNA template

The dNTPs add nucleotides down the length of the DNA single strands, thus literally copying the original double helix.

1988, a heat-resistant DNA polymerase isolated from bacteria inhabiting hot springs was purified and made commercially available. This so-called *"taq"* form of DNA polymerase allowed the development of the automatic PCR apparatus and with the growing awareness by scientists of what PCR could do, PCR was on the way to replacing other gene cloning methods.

Choosing from an impressive array of accomplishments in many areas of science and technology, the highly respected journal *Science* selected PCR as the major scientific development of 1989 and chose for its first "molecule of the year" the DNA polymerase that drives the reaction.

PCR has already had many valuable applications. One of the first uses of PCR led to diagnosis of sickle-cell anemia and later to the detection of the virus that causes AIDS. In cancer diagnosis, PCR can pinpoint which genes are turned on or off because the mRNA molecules coming from the gene can be converted into DNA sequences that then can be copied by PCR. Eventually most harmful genes will probably be determined by first cloning them by PCR, and because only minute amounts of starting material are needed, genetic screening can be done early. For example, in some *in vitro* fertilization clinics, tests are being done on cells from human embryos to search for certain hidden genetic defects before the embyro is implanted in the womb to develop into a "test-tube" baby.

Hitherto impossible developmental biology studies are beginning to be accomplished with PCR. This will enable scientists to study gene expression during embryo development. For example, activity of the dystrophin gene which is altered in Duchenne muscular dystrophy has been studied by PCR analysis of its DNA.

DNA in trace materials (blood, hair) found at the scene of a crime can be compared with DNA from suspects; both acquittals and convictions have resulted from this kind of comparison. Fascinating conclusions are being reached about the evolutionary relationships among humans based on PCR-amplified DNA.

For example, in 1990, by studying PCR-amplified DNA from many scattered groups of Native Americans, biologists traced the origin of all New World Native Americans to four women who were members of a small, intrepid band of Asian explorers who apparently migrated across the Bering land bridge to what is now Alaska some 20,000 years ago. Also in 1990, researchers using PCR traced the origins of modern humans to a tribe that lived in South Africa about 200,000 years ago.

Evolutionary biology now has a new and powerful tool. As the Human Genome Project adds to the DNA map, more direct and more accurate conclusions can be reached about the chronology of our origins and those of all other life as well. Svante Paabo, a biochemist at Berkeley, is among a new breed of "molecular archeologists." He has analyzed DNA from a 2400-year-old Egyptian mummy and a 7000-year-old human brain preserved in a Florida bog. He and others hope to draw genetic profiles of ancient peoples and compare them with modern humans to trace cultural as well as evolutionary lineages.

In addition to these fascinating applications of PCR, this remarkably simple method of cloning genes has become a critical component in the mapping and sequencing of the human genome.

*   *   *

What we have described with only a sampling of the jargon of molecular biology is, in less esoteric language, the fulfillment of the dreams of generations of scientists. The gene, final arbiter of all the functions of living creatures, has been located, removed, multiplied, purified, and awaits our bidding.

Would it have been possible, with the tools at our disposal, to have turned away from isolating and cloning human genes? Certainly not. The information generated by human gene cloning, mapping, and sequencing during the Human Genome Project will be the source book for human genetics in the twenty-first century and beyond. Let's look now at the heart of the Human Genome Project: the mapping and sequencing of human genes.

7

MAPS AND MARKERS

The search for our human genes begins, quite logically, with a map. Ordinary maps range from those indicating the landmarks of large areas to those more useful, detailed maps which guide the casual visitor to a new destination.

To map accurately the borders, highways, cities, and towns of a state requires that an enormous fund of information be available to the cartographer. To magnify a city's dimensions into a map of individual streets necessitates even more data. Chromosome mapping is the process of determining the relative position of genes or other recognizable landmarks on chromosomes, and requires information gleaned from both traditional genetics and molecular biology.

If one begins with a reference point such as a prominent building, a good city map will allow one to find a particular street. The establishment of recognizable landmarks on chromosomes can lead one to the location of specific genes on those chromosomes. The Human Genome Project has literally set out to develop maps which eventually will lead scientists to the location of every gene on all the human chromosomes (as well as the genes on several nonhuman genomes).

What would be the use of such maps? Is it really necessary to devote years of effort to attempt to determine the chromosomal sites of genes? Why not just isolate and study genes as individual units and construct a map later, if possible?

That sounds logical, but if we continue the map analogy we can see why such an objection, while seemingly plausible, is invalid. Remember that the human genome is a strand of DNA, 6 feet long in its unwound state, encompassing 50,000 to 100,000 genes. Just as it would be impossible to locate a particular house on a certain street in an unfamiliar city without the assistance of a map, so too we first need a chromosome map before we can determine even the approximate location of individual genes.

Showing the extraordinary utility of even an incomplete map of the chromosomes, preliminary maps of the human genome already constructed have allowed us to locate the genes linked to a variety of human diseases. As of August 1990, the relative position of almost 5000 genes had been located. Among them are the genes responsible for such devastating disorders as hemophilia, cystic fibrosis, sickle-cell anemia, and polycystic kidney disease.

The mapping of these genes has led in some cases to tests that diagnose a disease and allow detailed study of the causative gene that may lead to treatment or cure. It follows that as the resolution of gene maps increases we will be able to locate most of the thousands of genes that play a role in human disease.

Granted, a major impetus for gene mapping lies in its potential for improving human health. In addition, in the area of basic science, detailed understanding of the genome of humans as well as that of other species will deepen our insight into fundamental questions about genome organization, control of gene function, cell growth and development, and evolutionary biology. For example, why do our bodies age? Why are we allotted such a brief span of time before our cells and tissues wear out? Perhaps the genes will tell us.

Finally, maps are a *sine qua non* for determining the nitrogenous base sequence of the genome, the code spelling out the directions for life's activities. Once that code is obtained in its entirety, according to James Watson "we will be interpreting it a thousand years from now." By that he means that even knowing the sequence and location of the genes is only the first step. It must be followed by the lengthy process of determining the functions and interrelationships of those genes in the life of the human organism.

In order to explain mapping and its role under the aegis of the Human Genome Project, we will need to review briefly the topography and movements of the chromosomes to follow the logic behind mapping protocol.

You will recall that human cells each contain 46 chromosomes except for the sperm cells of the male and the mature egg cells of the female, each of which contains 23. The 46 chromosomes are actually in 23 pairs. Only one of these pairs helps to determine the sex of the human. The sex chromosomes are designated as XX in the female, XY in the male.

One member of each chromosome pair originates from the male parent (the paternal chromosome) of that individual and the other (the maternal chromosome) from the female parent. During the life of the cell the two members of each pair do not physically join. They are referred to as pairs, not because they are joined or identical, but because they are "homologous." That means that all along the length of the two chromosomes there are genes governing the same characteristic at the same position (locus) on each chromosome. Put simply, if the maternal chromosome has a gene for eye color at locus B, for example, then the paternal chromosome of that pair will also have a gene for eye color at that same position.

As we pointed out in our discussion of basic genetics these gene pairs, also called alleles, are not always identical genes. Both genes may be dominant, both may be recessive, or one may be dominant and the other recessive. You will recall that a recessive gene will ordinarily function only if the other member of the pair is also recessive, while a dominant gene will always function.

During cell division (mitosis), as one cell divides into two, each chromosome is copied, resulting in a total of 92 chromosomes, half of which move on to the new cell. When certain cells are transformed into sperm cells or egg cells, this doubling of chromosome numbers also takes place but there are two divisions of the cells. Therefore, from one original cell with 46 chromosomes, four cells (the gametes) are produced, each having 23 chromosomes. This reduction of chromosome number is critically important as a source of variability in inheritance because each gamete ends up with one of each of the original 23 pairs. Which one, whether of maternal or paternal origin, is a random event. Then, when the sperm and egg combine, an entirely unique combination of 46 chromosomes is formed, even though there are still 23 pairs.

Now comes the key to the traditional form of chromosome mapping. As strange as it may seem, in the early stages of sperm and egg produc-

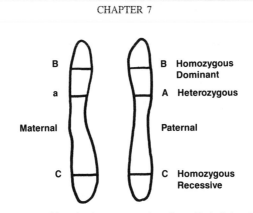

The genes—represented here by letters—are in pairs called alleles. These alleles are on the same position (locus) on a homologous chromosome pair.

tion, the chromosomes actually migrate within the nucleus so that each chromosome pair lines up side by side and the two members of the pair literally wrap around each other. No one knows what forces lure these partners to each other. After their tight but brief embrace they separate. In so doing they often interchange pieces in a process called "crossing-over." Amazingly, the chromosomes actually break and rejoin with pieces from the other member of the pair. If one chromosome were red and the other white, after crossing over and exchanging pieces both chromosomes would be part red and part white.

This disrupts the original order of the genes of each chromosome. We've already pointed out that the genes at the same specific site on both members of a chromosome pair are often different. This exchange of pieces between the members of these pairs creates chromosomes with new groups of genes, therefore adding another source of variability in the offspring. Remember, the child inherits only one member of each of the original 23 pairs of chromosomes.

The concept of the linear arrangement of genes on the chromosomes dates back to Mendel. However, the first experimental demonstration of crossing-over was performed by Alfred Sturtevant in 1913. Sturtevant produced the first chromosome map in which he calculated the relative

Mitosis **Meiosis**

(a) 46 diploid   46 diploid
       cell   cell

(b)   92   92

(c) 46   46   23 23 23 23
    diploid   haploid
     cells   gametes

(a) Each cell begins with 46 chromosomes. (b) The chromosomes replicate, resulting in 92 per cell. (c) In mitosis, the chromosomes are divided equally into two identical cells. In meiosis, there are two cell divisions, resulting in 4 gametes, each with 23 chromosomes. Each one of the latter chromosomes is a member of an original homologous pair.

positions of six genes including those for certain body colors and wing sizes on the X chromosome of the fruit fly, *Drosophila*. In this organism, as in humans, the female has two X chromosomes and the males have one X and one Y chromosome.

The kind of mapping which Sturtevant initiated and which is still being done today, albeit with more highly sophisticated techniques, is "genetic linkage" mapping. This type of map shows the arrangement of genes or other recognizable segments of DNA called "markers" along the chromosome. This map is constructed by taking advantage of the phenomenon of crossing-over. That simply means that if two genes, which we'll call A and B, are close together on the same chromosome, they ordinarily are inherited together. The only way that this would not happen is if that chromosome were to cross over with the other member of its pair, in this case at a point somewhere between A and B. Those two genes would then end up on separate chromosomes.

It stands to reason that the farther apart two genes are on a chromosome, the greater the chances that crossing-over can occur between them. If one can determine the frequency of crossing-over, one can put together a map which will indicate the relative positions of genes on a chromosome. Using such a map one cannot say "gene A is on this exact site on the chromosome." One can only say "Gene A is located far away from gene B but close to gene C, etcetera."

Since only one member of a chromosome pair normally ends up in a sperm or egg cell, then A and B will not be inherited together if crossing-over has occurred between them. Suppose that there is a way to detect the presence of A and B. One could look for these genes in the children, parents, or even the grandparents and trace the pattern of crossing-over in these generations. If this is done with a number of genes, then one ends up with a genetic linkage map. The distances between genes on a typical human genetic map are long. They average about ten million nitrogenous base pairs in length, which is roughly 5% of the size of a chromosome.

A limitation of genetic mapping is the need to trace specific genes or other DNA segments within several generations of a human family. Despite such difficulties, it was precisely the development of genetic mapping tools, made possible by the advent of molecular biology, that led to the feasibility of even contemplating the Human Genome Project.

In 1980, David Botstein of the California Institute of Technology pointed out that it might be possible to construct a complete linkage map of the human genome using restriction enzymes to cut up the chromosomes into patterns whose inheritance could be followed within families.

By 1987, when a partial map had already helped to narrow the search for several major diseases related to genes, the National Research Council (NRC) committee of the National Institutes of Health called for an immediate effort to develop a genetic linkage map as a goal of a concerted genome project.

Several members of the committee began with serious reservations about the usefulness of a special initiative in "genomics"—a term coined in 1986 by Thomas Roderick of the Jackson Laboratory in Bar Harbor, Maine to refer to the mapping, sequencing, and other processes of analysis of complex genomes. The term has survived in the title of the journal, *Genomics*, an international journal of gene mapping and sequencing, emphasizing analyses of human and other complex genomes. Despite the early doubts, the concept of a large-scale effort to create a complete map and sequence of the human genome within 15 years also survived as a unanimous recommendation.

The NRC committee recommended that researchers map first and sequence later for two reasons. First of all, rapid advances in mapping were anticipated because of new molecular techniques, while sequencing would require improvements in technology anticipated but not yet available. Second, having a map is essential to efficient sequencing.

The committee also recommended that technological developments should be stressed at the outset. Existing methods of mapping and sequencing were not sufficient to reach the announced goals in the proposed 15-year period. Also, they suggested that model nonhuman organisms be studied because of the value of such information for the analysis and understanding of the human genome.

A subsequent report from the Office of Technology Assessment in 1988 repeated the original recommendations regarding the mapping and sequencing of the genomes of human and other organisms. In an effort to curtail criticisms that the undertaking was too massive and unprecedented an effort they stated that "there is no single human genome project but instead many projects."

As it turned out, the attempt to portray this undertaking as a complex of diffuse but parallel series of programs was short-lived. As organizational meetings among the departments, agencies, and leading individuals proliferated, a consensus developed which is expressed succinctly in the title of the DOE/NIH five-year plan, released in February 1990. It reads, "Understanding Our Genetic Inheritance—the U.S. Human Genome Project: The First Five Years, Fiscal Year 1991–1995." According to the document, "a centrally coordinated project focused on specific objectives is believed to be the most efficient and least expensive way" to achieve the mapping and sequencing objectives.

Congress received these recommendations in February 1990 in response to its request for a report describing a comprehensive spending plan and optimal strategy for mapping and sequencing the human genome. In terms of mapping, the recommendations had become more specific. The goals, in language which we will decipher shortly, are stated as follows:

1. Complete a fully connected human genetic map with markers spaced an average of two to five centimorgans apart. Identify each marker by an STS.

2. Assemble STS maps of all human chromosomes with the goal of having markers spaced at approximately one hundred thousand [nitrogenous] base pair intervals.

3. Generate overlapping sets of cloned DNA or closely spaced unambiguously ordered markers with continuity over lengths of two million base pairs for large parts of the human genome.

What are the meanings of these new terms, centimorgans and STS? How are these ambitious goals to be met? We need to look a bit more closely at mapping to answer these questions.

Goal one refers to the construction of a detailed genetic linkage map. As we have explained, such a map uses the frequency of crossing-over as a measure of the distance between two genes or other detectable DNA segments. A crossover rate of 1% between two sites on a chromosome has been arbitrarily designated as equal to one "map unit." Thus two genes on the same chromosome are said to be ten map units apart if experiments show a 10% crossover frequency between them. This map unit is expressed as one centimorgan, or cM, in honor of the great geneticist Thomas Hunt Morgan.

This method of mapping tends to give an inaccurate map distance between genes that are a long way apart because multiple crossovers between them will often occur. The most accurate genetic linkage maps are those for which observations have been made on the crossover values between as many different sites on the chromosome as possible.

Using the data from laboratory crosses made among over 1000 generations of *Drosophila*, the genetic linkage map of the fruit fly is one of the most complete for any organism with the exception of the bacterium *E. coli*. We have excellent maps as well for laboratory mice, corn, and *Neurospora*. Obviously, planned genetic crosses are not possible in humans and the number of offspring from any one mating is relatively small. Compared to a life span of two weeks for *Drosophila*, the period of time required for another generation to occur in humans typically allows under the best of conditions three generations for study, the children, parents, grandparents. As a result, until very recently, relatively few human genes had been placed on a genetic linkage map and most of those were on the X chromosome.

It is easy to see why the X chromosome lends itself to mapping. Crossing-over between X chromosomes can take place only in the female since she is XX. The male X and Y chromosomes are only partly homologous. They are the only human chromosome pair which differ greatly in size, the Y being much smaller. As a result there are many genes on the larger X chromosome which do not have a corresponding gene on the Y. Therefore, even if a gene on the X chromosome is recessive, it could still be active because there would be no possibility of a dominant gene on the Y to repress its activity. Hemophilia and certain forms of color blindness, which occur almost exclusively in males, are classic examples of genes which are obviously on the X chromosome because of this inheritance pattern. Such disorders are possible in females only if both X chromosomes bear the same recessive genes, a very rare occurrence.

We have already pointed out that the closer together genes are on the same chromosome, the less frequently crossing-over takes place between them. Therefore, rather than trying to follow the inheritance of only entire genes, one can estimate the distance between a gene of particular interest and any other DNA sequence that is identifiable (a "marker") on the same chromosome. This procedure is very important because the major problem in genetic linkage lies in detecting the presence of the genes in a person's cells. This identification is made easier if one is following genes which cause a detectable genetic disease. These genes can be followed over several generations if the symptoms of the disease are obvious.

Let's look at a practical example of the use of a marker. If people who develop a genetic disease almost always inherit the same version of a certain marker, the disease gene and the marker must lie very close together on the same chromosome. Correlating the marker and the disease gene requires that two conditions be met. First, the marker must be detectable, and second, it must be found in several distinguishable forms. If the two forms of the marker on the chromosome pair are identical, then crossovers between the diseased gene and the marker would be untraceable in the offspring. To use a fanciful hypothesis, suppose that the disease gene were near to a purple marker. If the corresponding site on the other member of that chromosome pair were also purple, then an exchange between those two sites by a crossing-over would result in both chromosomes having a purple site. If the corresponding site was not purple but yellow, a crossover would be readily detectable.

Until recently, only a few markers met such stringent criteria. The first assignment of a gene to a specific non-sex chromosome occurred in 1968 when scientists showed that the inheritance of certain blood group proteins was linked to chromosome number 1. Only a few dozen such markers were then known and for want of such markers most of the human genome remained inaccessible.

It should be stressed here that the decision to map the human genome actually occurred long before the current large-scale coordinated initiative. The scientist who had the most influence in those early years was Victor McCusick of Johns Hopkins University. In 1968 he began to put together his book *The Mendelian Inheritance of Man*. In 1971, there were 15 genes that had been mapped to human chromosomes. The ninth and latest edition in 1990, still being compiled and edited by McCusick, lists 4937 mapped genes.

In the late 1960s, even before the molecular biology breakthroughs of the next decade, a fascinating method was developed that expanded the possibility of correlating specific genes with particular chromosomes. The technique uses human and rodent cells grown in culture.

It also involves the use of a virus with a most useful property. Most viruses have a specific point for attachment to a cell. A "Sendai" virus has several points of attachment so that it can simultaneously attach to two different cells if they are close together. A virus is so small compared to the average cell that this attachment to two very closely adjacent cells often causes the membranes of the two cells to fuse together and the two cells blend into one. If suspensions of mouse tumor cells and human connective tissue cells are mixed together in the presence of Sendai virus, the virus may cause the formation of human–mouse hybrid cells. The old question "Are you a man or a mouse?" can now be answered by "Both."

When viewed through a microscope, human and mouse chromosomes can be easily told apart.

Fortunately for the experimental technique, the human chromosomes are gradually eliminated from the cells as the hybrid cells divide. Careful manipulation of this characteristic can result in a population of cells that contains one or even part of one human chromosome. Eventually, cell lines can be developed that contain, in total, all of the human chromosomes. In studying such cells therefore, one can then look for human DNA which is not ordinarily found in mouse cells. The presence of such DNA in a hybrid cell means that it has actually become part of the genome. Of the approximately 5000 human genes mapped so far, about 1000 have been located by this process of making hybrid cells.

The Sendai virus had put new life into genome mapping, but despite this ingenious approach its use was still limited to assigning some genes to certain chromosomes, somewhat analogous to determining that a particular city is in a specific country.

The recombinant DNA revolution of the 1970s supplied the tools to bring about unprecedented advances in genetic linkage mapping. Recognizing the potential of the new molecular approach, in 1978 Raymond White of the University of Utah committed his lab to developing a set of markers based on the detection of unique DNA sequences.

He and others soon developed a strategy which led to the possibility of mapping human genes on the scale envisioned by the Human Genome Project. It is based on the normal variation between nitrogenous base sequences in chromosome pairs. A difference in these sequences between the two chromosomes occurs, on the average, every 200 to 500 base pairs.

You will recall that restriction enzymes cut nucleotides at specific nitrogenous base sequences. That means that a variation in DNA sequence that creates or eliminates a site where an enzyme will cut will alter the length of some of the DNA fragments when that DNA is treated with the enzyme. This variation between restriction enzyme cutting sites between the same areas of chromosome pairs creates a "restriction–fragment length polymorphism" (RFLP) (pronounced riflips by the in crowd). This formidable-sounding phenomenon has moved genetic linkage mapping to a new era. RFLPs provide an enormously rich supply of detectable markers.

If we are looking at an entire human genome, however, a typical restriction enzyme has millions of cutting sites to work on. How can one or a few fragments of different sizes be located among millions which are the same? The answer lies once again in the use of gel electrophoresis. The cut fragments of the genome are spread out on a gel according to size. Then a DNA probe can be applied to pick out a specific spot in the assortment of fragments.

If the radioactive bands appear at different places on gel patterns of DNA from different individuals, the DNA probe has detected a variation in the enzyme cutting pattern between the DNA of those two individuals. Many hundreds of probes may have to be screened before a usable one is found. When a probe is found, one then has a powerful marker system— the probe and the RFLP that it detects. The inheritance pattern of the RFLP can then be traced instead of relying on tracing a disease. RFLPs are scattered abundantly throughout the human genome and have multiplied manyfold the markers available for mapping our chromosomes.

RFLPs have been a useful tool in providing a definitive diagnosis for a variety of diseases including sickle-cell anemia and Huntington's disease. In addition to diagnosis, the linkage between a marker such as an RFLP and a disease gene is the first critical step in narrowing down the search for that gene and a means of isolating large amounts of a specific chromosomal segment for the purpose of isolating and characterizing the gene itself.

A person's individual set of RFLP markers can be used to produce a "genetic fingerprint." These have proven to be very useful in forensic medicine since the probability that two people would have the same set of RFLP markers is infinitesimally small. The courts now accept evidence based on identification of individuals through such analysis of DNA.

Scientists estimate that 3000 well-spaced markers will be needed to achieve a completely linked map with markers an average of one centimorgan apart. Each centimorgan covers about 30 to 40 genes. For the first five years of the Human Genome Project the goal has been set as the development of a map in which markers are separated by a minimum of two to five centimorgans, which would require 600 to 1500 markers. To have markers at even intervals on the chromosomes, however, requires a much larger set of random markers on the map. Also, DNA must be

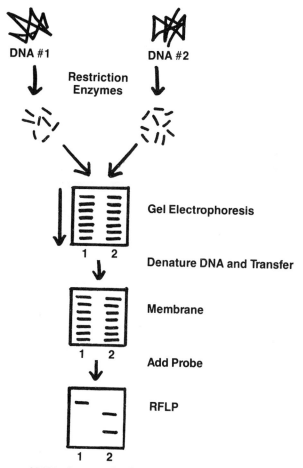

The pattern of DNA pieces cut by the same restriction enzymes varies with the source of the DNA. The variation (RFLP) is seen in the rates of travel along an electrophoresis gel due to the different size of the fragments.

collected from hundreds of individuals in dozens of large families and tested for the RFLP characteristics of each marker site.

A recent innovation has made RFLP use even more effective. At many sites on the human chromosome DNA has simple base sequences that do not code for proteins and are repeated many times. The origin and significance of these "tandem repeats" is a mystery but they have proven to be of great use in linkage mapping. The number of repeats at a given locus can vary from a few to hundreds of copies. If a restriction enzyme cuts near these variable tandem repeats, the resulting fragments will vary correspondingly in length. This variable number of tandem repeats (VNTRs) is so common that the odds are good that an individual will carry different versions of them on homologous chromosomes.

Even newer methods of mapping have been recently developed. In 1988, David Cox and Richard Myers of the University of California at San Francisco announced that they had devised a totally new approach to genetic linkage mapping which they termed "radiation hybrid mapping." Instead of looking at how often two markers are separated during crossing-over, their method looks at how often the markers are broken apart if the chromosomes are bombarded with X rays. Early trials have shown that this approach may lead to a 20-fold greater resolution than current linkage mapping.

While the genetic linkage map provides a powerful tool for narrowing the search for genes, it is not sufficient for actually isolating a gene and removing it for study. That kind of specificity must come from a second approach, "physical mapping." The physical map provides the real physical distance between landmarks on the chromosomes. In discussing the physical map, we need to explain the concept of STS, the use of which applies to physical as well as genetic mapping.

Physical mapping depends on the complex and difficult task of attempting to determine the exact order in which the pieces of DNA that are being analyzed had originally existed in the chromosome. The distance between sites on a chromosome is measured in terms of physical length such as numbers of nucleotide pairs. The ultimate physical map would be the exact order of the 3 billion nitrogenous bases in the nucleotides that constitute the human genome.

Physical maps can be put together in a variety of ways, some of which date back to the early years of human genetic analysis while others take advantage of the most recent developments of molecular biology. There are two major categories of physical maps. The first is the "cytogenetic" map which displays a pattern of landmarks that are actually visible on the chromosomes. Here, the inheritance of genes is linked to the inheritance of areas on the chromosomes that can be seen through the microscope.

A variety of staining techniques have been developed which highlight certain regions or "bands" in the chromosomes. Each of the 46 chromosomes turns out to have a unique intricate banding pattern. The molecular basis of these bands, which occur in other organisms as well, is not known. They are presumed to be due to the folding produced by the interaction of DNA and proteins. A single band represents about 10 million base pairs. Nearly 1000 bands have been detected in the human chromosomes by staining and light microscopy. A single band represents an average of 100 genes.

A standardized map of bands in human chromosomes has been developed which has proven to be useful in correlating visible, often subtle changes in chromosome structure in certain genetic disorders. For example, some cancers are associated with the production of abnormal DNA sequences which appear as changes in band patterns. Also, the detection of a "deletion," the loss of a small part of a chromosome, is aided by looking for losses of bands.

A typical example is seen in the diagnosis of the deletion of a piece of chromosome number 5, which occurs in "cri-du-chat" syndrome, marked by severe mental retardation. Even though there is relatively little detailed genetic information to be derived from following banding patterns compared to the diagnostic capabilities which result from more sophisticated mapping, it remains for now a very valuable tool, particularly for prenatal diagnosis.

An innovative extension of the cytogenetic approach was developed in 1970 by Mary Lou Pardue and Joseph Gall. It has since been modified to allow one literally to visualize the location of a specific DNA sequence on a chromosome. This technique involves preparing a karyotype (chromosomes spread out on a slide) so that the DNA in the chromosomes can be made into single strands and exposed to a radioactive DNA probe. The probe will bind as usual with its complementary DNA sequence. Exposing the slide to a photographic emulsion for weeks or even months results in the areas of probe binding being detectable as dark spots on the chromosomes. This has been a very productive approach to physically mapping many genes and other DNA markers to specific chromosomes but it still can only pinpoint the actual location to within about 10 million base pairs.

A recent refinement reported in 1989 improves upon that resolution. Rather than use radioactive DNA as a probe, David Ward and Peter Lichter labeled the probe with a "reporter" molecule, a small molecule to which certain proteins can attach. For example, in a common form of this approach the vitamin biotin is attached to a small DNA probe and the probe is applied to the chromosomes. Then the chromosome spread is incubated with fluorescent "avidin," a protein which binds wherever it finds biotin. The biotin–avidin complex shows up as a bright, yellow-green dot on the chromosome. This can be done within hours as compared to the method which uses radioactivity.

A second category of physical map is a highly detailed map which is made by putting together complete sets of pieces of DNA. These pieces of DNA are cut out by restriction enzymes from individual chromosomes, groups of chromosomes, or the entire genome and then cloned. Theoretically, all of the separate cloned pieces linked together in the correct order will reconstruct the original DNA.

That is easier said than done. The problem lies in recreating the original order of these segments so that they are once again in the same order as they were before being separated. Try cutting up a piece of string (a chromosome) into thousands of pieces (fragments made by restriction enzymes). Now mix them all together and reassemble them in their original order. Impossible? Of course it is. But wait, there is something we didn't tell you. The very places where you cut the string were a different color than the rest of the string. That means, for example, if you cut through a red area in the string, then all you have to do is find two red ends and reconnect them. That at least will give you a clue as to how some of the pieces relate. Simple enough with colored string, but what about chromosome fragments?

Well, the fragments are not different colors, but they do have differences among their DNA sequences. How could we use this to recreate the original order of these segments? The answer lies in making "contigs." These are DNA fragments that are contiguous (next to and touching) to each other in the chromosome and are related to one another not by a direct end-to-end connection but by a partial overlap. Picture contigs as dominoes. Placed on end, a row of dominoes, when the first is pushed over, will fall into a sequence of slightly overlapping pieces.

How can one possibly find out the order of these contigs along the original DNA as well as determine which end of the string of contigs lies at which end of the chromosome? First, clones of the DNA fragments are made. Then one tries to identify which clones have some overlapping DNA sequences. This is again done by using gel electrophoresis.

The resulting pattern of many fragment sizes is observed along the length of the gel. If two clones contain overlapping segments of DNA, then a portion of the spots on the gel pattern will also overlap. For example, a contig would be discovered if clone A contained fragments a–b–c and clone B contained fragments b–c–d. The overlapping of b and c would link clone B to the end of clone A.

In contig mapping one begins with DNA that has broken into many pieces and attempts to put them back in order. If the pieces are 30 to 50 kilobases (kb) long, as they frequently are in human gene clones, it would take more than 1000 pieces arranged end to end to complete the map of the shortest chromosome. This problem is being alleviated in part by the use of YACs (yeast artificial chromosomes) which can clone DNA of up to 500 kb. There is also increasing use of fluorescent reporter molecules, mentioned earlier in connection with genetic linkage mapping, which in this case are bound to pieces of the contigs. The visible labeled spots make the relative position of two contigs easy to see.

In addition, there are novel techniques still in developmental stages which hold out great promise in mapping. One of the problems with restriction enzymes is that they recognize a specific base sequence of a maximum of eight bases. The larger the genome, the more often those particular sequences will appear. In the human genome, that adds up to about 50,000 times.

What is needed is a restriction enzyme that recognizes a longer strand—perhaps 15 to 20 bases. But nature does not make such enzymes. An innovative technique to get around this dilemma was reported in August 1988 for plasmid DNA and in June 1990 for yeast chromosomes by Michael Koob and Waclaw Szybalski of the University of Wisconsin. It is a unique way to modify DNA to "cover" all but one of the cutting sites for the restriction enzyme use. They called it the "Achilles' heel cleavage." If applied successfully to the human genome, the technique could break the chromosomes into manageable chunks which could be sequenced more easily.

Another development vital to the Human Genome Project in relation to mapping is the ingenious technique of "flow-sorting" of chromosomes. In 1975, Jay W. Gray and his colleagues at the Lawrence Livermore National Laboratory reported that suspensions of fluorescent-stained chromosomes could be analyzed at a rate of several thousand per second and purified and sorted based on their fluorescence intensity. In 1979, human chromosomes were first purified by this flow-sorting, a separation which has been periodically improved to the point where triple-laser high-speed sorting routinely separates most human chromosomes.

As a result of the ability to separate large numbers of human chromosomes, both the Lawrence Livermore and the Los Alamos National Laboratories began to receive requests from scientists who wanted a supply of individual chromosome groups for analysis. As a result, the National Laboratory Gene Library Project (NLGLP), financed by the Office of Health and Environmental Research of the U.S. Department of Energy, was founded in 1983. Beginning with flow-sorted chromosomes, this facility produces DNA libraries for use in studying the molecular biology of genes, studying and diagnosing genetic diseases, and constructing physical maps of chromosomes. So far over 2300 libraries and other materials have been distributed by the NLGLP to many laboratories that could not afford to produce these themselves.

A major difficulty frequently facing those trying to assemble physical maps of chromosomes has been the inability to compare the results of one mapping technique with those of another or to combine maps derived from different techniques into a single map. In September 1989, Maynard

V. Olson, Leroy Hood, Charles Cantor, and David Botstein, all members of the original NRC Committee on Mapping and Sequencing the Human Genome, published a proposal entitled "Common Language for Physical Mapping of the Human Genome." They proposed that data from all physical mapping procedures be reported in a common "language."

In this protocol, each particular segment of DNA that had been put onto a map would be identified as unique by what they called a "sequence tagged site," or STS. This would be the nitrogenous base sequence of a short stretch within the DNA under study. About 200 to 500 base pairs of sequence would be sufficient, an amount which is quite readily determined. This STS would become an entry in an STS data base, which would store the sequence information. What would be the advantage of this STS system?

If the specific goals of physical mapping are to be met within the proposed five-year period, physical mapping data must be compiled on long continuous stretches of DNA. With the STS approach, researchers could use whatever mapping techniques they wished; however, results would always be reported in terms of the STS markers. Each mapped DNA section would be defined by a short DNA sequence within it that occurs only once in the genome. Basically, it would involve determining a short DNA sequence and then using this sequence to make primers for the polymerase chain reaction discussed in Chapter 6. The use of these primers would then allow anyone in a reasonably equipped laboratory to make millions of copies of the STS DNA sequence in a few hours by using PCR.

In fact, with the STS sequence stored electronically in a central data base, there would be no need to obtain a probe or other material from the original researcher. Knowing the sequence, one could make PCR primers and regenerate the STS for analysis in one's own laboratory. The STS system will provide a common language and common landmarks for mapping, reduce costs, and will allow genetic and physical maps to be cross-referenced.

Let's reflect for a moment on an underlying theme in the current chapter. There is a mind-set among scientists which is exemplified on a grand scale in the initiators of and leading participants in the Human Genome Project. It is an unbridled optimism that, despite seemingly intractable problems, ever newer technological developments will arise to solve those very difficulties.

What might seem like blind faith is, in fact, a *modus operandi* which has stimulated the impressive scientific developments of our current era. It is an attitude that has served the scientific community well. In the present case, the scientists instrumental in giving birth to and nurturing the Human Genome Project quite frankly admitted in the mid-1980s and continue to admit freely at meetings and in their publications that the Human Genome Project will not be completed without a quantum leap forward in the technology of genetic analysis.

In San Diego, California in October 1989, at "Human Genome I," the first in a series of annual international conferences held to report on the progress of the Human Genome Project, the 900 attendees were told that the success of the proposed 15-year project would require a five- to tenfold improvement in technology for the first five years and another five- to tenfold improvement in the next five. There was a consensus that this was possible.

Is this kind of optimism naive? Not if one considers that since the members of the National Research Council Committee assembled in 1986 to make recommendations that originated this undertaking, pulsed-field gel electrophoresis, yeast artificial chromosome cloning, fluorescent labels, radiation hybrid mapping, chromosome flow-sorting, and Achilles' heel cleavage have all been either invented or upgraded significantly. Innovative techniques have arrived to meet the needs of ever more detailed genetic analysis.

Regardless of whether or not quantities of DNA are made available by the now "classic" method of gene cloning with bacteria or by the newer magic of PCR, the problem of determining the ultimate code of life in the nitrogenous base sequence of DNA remains. The DOE/NIH five-year plan goals relative to DNA sequencing are as follows:

1. (To) improve current methods and/or develop new methods for DNA sequencing that will allow large-scale sequencing of DNA at a cost of 50 cents per base pair.

2. Determine the sequence of an aggregate of 10 million base pairs

of human DNA in large continuous stretches in the course of technology development and validation.

3. Sequence an aggregate of about 20 million base pairs of DNA from a variety of model organisms focusing on stretches that are 1 million base pairs long in the course of the development and validation of new and/or improved DNA sequencing technology.

We have in the sequencing goals of the HGP yet another example of faith in the advance of technology. The goals call for a significant increase in the speed and cost of sequencing which science has not yet achieved. The practical problem in efficiently determining the precise sequence of the 3 billion bases in the human genome is one of scale.

In 1953, when James Watson and Francis Crick described the double-helical structure of DNA, there was no convenient way to sequence even the shortest of DNA molecules. By the early 1970s, it took about one year to work out 10 to 20 base pairs of sequence—hardly the pace at which one would approach the human genome.

The scene changed when Frederick Sanger turned his attention to the problem. Sanger, already renowned for being the first ever to determine the complete amino acid sequence of a protein (insulin) in 1953, devised the first of several direct DNA sequencing methods in 1975. With this technique the base pair sequence of a small bacterial virus was quickly determined. Its nucleotide sequence codes for just nine proteins.

An equally effective method was developed in 1977 at Harvard University by Alan Maxam and Walter Gilbert. It was based on the chemical breakdown of DNA fragments. Soon the 5226 base pairs of an animal virus, simian virus SV40, was determined, as well as the 4632 base pairs of a bacterial plasmid. It became possible for a single worker to determine the sequence of up to 5000 nitrogenous bases in one year, a major improvement but still insufficient to consider the human genome as a feasible subject for sequencing. By 1990 it would be possible for an individual to generate about 2000 bases of sequence per day. What were the reasons for this quantum leap?

The advance resulted from a series of modifications to the Sanger and the Maxam and Gilbert methods and, very importantly, automation.

So far, the only complete DNA sequences that have been recorded are those of the viruses, the longest being that of cytomegalovirus, which has 250,000 base pairs. Many others, including that of our own genome, are under intense study.

What are these techniques that are allowing us to discover our genetic code, about which James Watson has written, "A more important set of instruction books will never be found by human beings"? Modifications of both Sanger's method and that of Maxam and Gilbert are now widely used with the former now favored for large-scale DNA sequence determination.

The Sanger method is based on some of the same principles that led the PCR technique. A section of a DNA double helix is first separated to form single strands. These are placed into each of four test tubes. Each portion is incubated with all the ingredients necessary for the formation of new complementary strands: a radioactively labeled oligo primer, the enzyme DNA polymerase, and all four dNTPs—dATP, dGTP, dCTP, and dTTP. Each mixture also contains a different one of the four ddNTPs: ddATP, ddGTP, ddCTP, and ddTTP.

Just as in PCR, a new single strand is synthesized by adding dNTPs one at a time, beginning with the primer, continuing until a ddNTP joins the growing strand. This stops any further addition of the dNTP nucleotides. Since the dNTPs and the ddNTPs are both in the mixture, they are, in a sense, competing for the chance to be incorporated in the growing

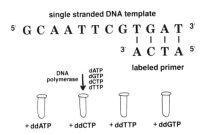

In the Sanger method, single-stranded DNA with an attached primer is put into each of the four tubes with the indicated ingredients.

single stranded DNA template

⁵' **G C A A T T C G T G A T** ³'
               | | | | |
new strand ends   ³' **C A C T A** ⁵'

          ddCTP   primer

new strand ends   ³' **G C A C T A** ⁵'

          ddGTP   primer

new strand ends   ³' **A G C A C T A** ⁵'

          ddATP   primer

Strand synthesis ends whenever a ddNTP attaches.

DNA strand. Since there are typically millions of DNA sections in the original sample, the odds are that a whole set of new strands of varying lengths will be made, each terminated when a ddNTP adds on instead of a dNTP.

The newly synthesized DNA strands in each of the four separate reaction mixtures are separated from each other by polyacrylamide gel electrophoresis. These gels are so precise that it is possible, for example, to clearly distinguish a DNA fragment 600 bases in length from one 601 in length. The sequence of the new strands can be read directly from the spots on the gel.

The spots are detectable because of the presence of the radioactively labeled primer. The sequence of the original DNA can be deduced in the following manner. By starting at the top of the electrophoresis gel where the smallest, lightest fragments have migrated and then recording the band with the next shortest chain and so on, one can read the sequence of the synthesized DNA by following the growing length of nucleotides. This, of course, will actually be the complement of the original DNA strand.

For sequencing on a smaller scale, one can utilize a different approach. In the Maxam and Gilbert method, the starting point is also a

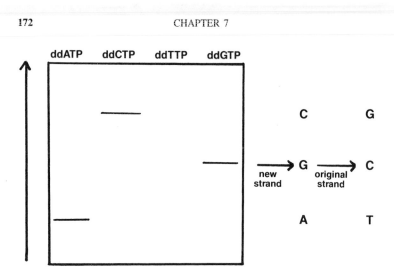

DNA fragments from the Sanger method on an electrophoresis gel. In an actual
sequencing procedure there would be hundreds of these bands on one gel. The
arrow indicates the direction of migration of the fragments. The sequence of the
newly synthesized strand can be read from the gel, from which can be inferred the
sequence of the complementary original strand.

collection of DNA single strands but in this method the 5′ end of each of
these strands is labeled with a radioactive form of phosphorus called ^{32}P.

The DNA is then treated briefly with a chemical that alters one of the
four nitrogenous base types, A, G, C, or T. Treatment with another
chemical agent will cut the strand at that point on the 5′ side of the
nucleotide, one, for example, containing adenine. Because the treatment
is brief, not all the adenine sites will be cut. This leaves some of the
original DNA fragments unbroken and also produces DNA pieces with all
possible fragment lengths which extend to each A site.

Three more samples of the DNA are now treated with the same

^{32}P $^{5′}$ T G T A C C A G G A T G $^{3′}$

single stranded DNA template

This single-stranded DNA is labeled with radioactive phosphorus on its 5′ end.

^{32}P $^{5'}$ **T G T A C C A G G** $^{3'}$

^{32}P $^{5'}$ **T G T A C C** $^{3'}$ cut at A

^{32}P $^{5'}$ **T G T** $^{3'}$ cut at A

The radioactively labeled single-stranded DNA is cut at the A sites.

procedure but with chemicals that break the DNA chain in each batch at one of the other three nitrogenous bases, in this case, G, C, or T. The mixture of pieces is then separated by electrophoresis with each treatment run on a separate gel lane.

The relative position of each spot on the gel indicates how many nucleotides are in the components of that spot because, of course, the smallest pieces migrate the farthest on the gel. The results of reading the gel are a direct index of the DNA sequence.

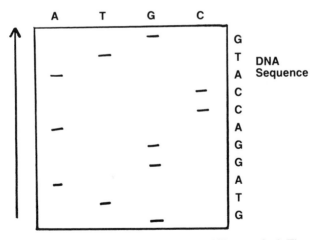

A gel electrophoresis pattern using the Maxam and Gilbert method. The arrow indicates the direction of migration of the DNA fragments. The sequence can be read directly.

However straightforward and logical the sequencing procedures might seem, it remains a daunting prospect to apply them to large genomes such as that of the human. In addition to the extreme length of such DNA molecules, there remains the requirement that the sections of the genome that are sequenced eventually be put into the same order in which they originally existed in the chromosome. This is where having a detailed physical map becomes of critical importance.

The problem facing the HGP, then, is to sequence DNA molecules at a rate which will meet the announced goals. As the five-year plan expresses it, "A substantial increase in the speed and reduction of cost of sequencing technology will be required." This is yet another example of how goals have been set without the means immediately at hand to achieve those goals. It is also another example of how advances have been made to at least begin to meet the demands of the occasion.

In the case of sequencing, a major improvement has been the development of an alternate method of detecting DNA in gels. Instead of radioactive labels, fluorescent tags can be applied. These are molecules that respond with a characteristic color when stimulated by a light from a source such as a laser. With fluorescence, where a variety of colors is possible, one can place a different fluorescent tag on each of the four sets of DNA fragments.

The use of fluorescent indicators has led to the crucial step of permitting DNA sequencing to be automated. In the late 1980s, while the planning for the HGP was already underway, several automated sequencing systems were developed which arrived just in time to make the idealistic goals of human genome sequencing seem much more feasible. The chemistry of attaching fluorophores (fluorescent chemicals) was developed sufficiently in 1986 to allow Lloyd Smith at the University of Wisconsin to develop an automated sequencer which works as follows.

One of four different fluorophores is attached to the primer used in the Sanger sequencing method. A different fluorophore is used in each of the four reactions. After the reactions are complete, the products are combined and electrophoresed on a single lane of a polyacrylamide gel. There is a light-sensitive fluorescent detector near the bottom of the gel which detects the fluorescent bands of DNA as they move by and determines their color. The DNA sequence is determined by the order of the bands as they pass by the detector. The bands with the smallest fragments will move by first, the next largest second, and so on. The detector data are stored and analyzed by microcomputer to yield the DNA sequence.

There are several aspects of the process of automated sequencing where improvements can increase its speed and efficiency. First, the extraordinarily timely advent of PCR has already simplified the cloning of the DNA needed to begin the sequencing procedure. PCR itself quickly became an automated procedure. The sequencing itself can be improved in several areas such as gel technology, detection sensitivity, development of more sensitive dyes, or modification of the light source which excites the fluorophores. For example, the use of ultrathin slab gels may allow high resolution that will detect bands containing DNA of above 1000 bases in length. Thin gels also dissipate heat more effectively and so permit higher voltages that result in faster separation. Also, improved automatic gel readers and sensitive cameras are under development to improve the conversion of images to computerized data.

The so-called "back end" of sequencing involves the computer hardware and software needed to acquire, analyze, cross-check, and integrate the hundreds or thousands of sets of data generated in the analyses. As a rule, the shorter the fragments being read, the more accurate the sequencing data. These data must be processed by computers to recognize overlaps so that the entire sequence can be assembled in the correct order. This is being addressed by the development and testing of new computer programs as well as the application of improvements in chip technology.

It was the consensus of those gathered at the first annual Genome Sequencing Conference in October 1989 that changes in DNA sequencing technology were more likely to be made by step-by-step improvements in the then-current technology than by instituting totally new technologies. However, in the five-year plan, released in February 1990, the position of the leaders of the HGP was that, regardless of the improvements that had been or would probably be made in automated detection of DNA sequences, it was by no means certain that such enhancements would bring down the cost of sequencing sufficiently.

In order to keep the costs of the HGP within the project's budgetary constraints, the cost of the automated processes and the handling procedures before and after it will have to be reduced to well below 50 cents per base pair. In early 1990, routine sequencing was estimated to cost $5 per base pair with the most advanced laboratories reporting a cost of $1–2 per base pair. In 1995, the cost of sequencing will be assessed and sequencing the entire human genome will not be considered unless that level has been reached.

As a result, entirely new approaches to DNA sequencing are being actively explored. These so-called "revolutionary" techniques are diverse in their principles and instrumentation. Among others, these include a method which is independent of the application of all traditional biochemical methods. Scanning tunneling microscopy (STM) was introduced in January 1989 as a result of collaboration between Lawrence Berkeley Laboratory and Lawrence Livermore National Laboratory. A tiny probe scans the DNA with the objective of distinguishing among the four bases on the sugar–phosphate backbone. Also, development of intense laser X-ray sources and high-quality X-ray optics may result in an analysis that could diagnose base sequences and produce enough data to reconstruct a holographic image of the molecule.

With these revolutionary schemes in progress, prediction of what form the ultimate technology for DNA sequencing will take is impossible. In order to assess progress and coordinate research on sequencing technology, the DOE Human Genome Program and the NIH National Center for Human Genome Research organized a Joint Working Group for DNA Sequencing. The group, consisting of members from academia and industry, met for the first time in May 1990.

Historically, high-resolution mapping and sequencing of entire genomes has focused on nonhuman organisms and viruses. Most of the technologies used in analysis of human chromosomes has been developed from work on other organisms. The genomes of organisms that are smaller and less complex than that of humans have been ideal systems for the development and testing of procedures needed for the analysis of the more complex human genome.

These organisms have also served as model systems for the many genetic and biochemical pathways which are common to all organisms.

For example, if two genes are located on the same chromosome in rodents such as the mouse, it is likely that those genes are also linked in humans. At least 33 of the same linked groups of genes have already been found in both mice and humans.

Usually, when attempting to determine the role of a gene, the first step is to look for similarities between its DNA sequence and those of genes from other organisms. For example, yeast has a number of genes identical to or very similar to those of humans. Fruit flies have been shown to contain a DNA sequence which determines the expression of particular groups of genes during its development. The same, almost identical sequence has been found in humans.

Particularly relevant in this regard is the mouse genome. It consists of 3 billion base pairs and has been especially useful for comparisons because of the many biological similarities between the mouse and the human. The five-year plan includes, among the other goals listed earlier, that of preparing "a genetic map of the mouse genome based on DNA markers, [and] start[ing] physical mapping on one or two chromosomes." This will lead to the development of a physical map that can be directly compared with the human physical map.

The mapping and sequencing of several other organisms is well underway. It is expected that the full sequence of *E. coli*'s estimated 4.7 million base pairs, already one third completed, will be available by 1994. By mid-1990, the use of yeast artificial chromosomes had enabled researchers to map approximately half of the *Drosophila* genome.

Another intriguing undertaking involves *Caenorhabditis elegans*— a tiny nematode, or roundworm. Laboratories in the U.S. and the U.K. have begun the sequencing of the 100 million base pairs of its genome, roughly the size of an average human chromosome. The biology of this little worm has been thoroughly studied. It is known to have exactly 958 cells and each cell division during development has been carefully traced. Relating its genomic sequence to such unprecedented knowledge of a multicelled organism should prove extraordinarily useful in correlating gene structure with gene function.

In the 1960s and 1970s when DNA was first analyzed in terms of its base sequence, there was little need for sophisticated data storage and retrieval systems to record the experimental results. With the methods of that time very little sequencing could be accomplished. Gene mapping had accumulated far more data than sequencing efforts. For mapping data there was the atlas, available since 1966, which listed the approximate location of genes that had been traced by their inheritance pattern— *Mendelian Inheritance in Man* edited by Victor McCusick of Johns Hopkins University.

Since 1986, the Howard Hughes Medical Institute (HHMI) has supported the computerization of McCusick's list. In 1990, Johns Hopkins University established the "Genome Data Base" (GDB) designed to collect, organize, store, and distribute genetic mapping information. It also serves as a repository for genetic disease information applicable to patient care. Currently, the other major data base relative to mapping is the "Human Gene Mapping Library" (HGML) located in New Haven, Connecticut at the Yale–Howard Hughes Medical Institute.

When the revolution in sequencing techniques arrived in the late 1970s, an obvious need developed for data bases containing the sequence information about the origin of the sequences submitted and a variety of other related data. The National Science Foundation (NSF) sponsored a workshop at Rockefeller University to discuss the development of DNA sequence data bases and subsequent meetings included the sponsorship of NIH and the European Molecular Biology Laboratory (EMBL).

The eventual outcome was the establishment of the EMBL Data Library in Heidelberg and the GenBank data base at the Los Alamos National Laboratory. Each of these now carries sequence data and related information for the human genome as well as bacteria, yeast, fruit fly, mouse, and other genomes.

A third repository of such data is the DNA Data Bank of Japan (DDBJ) at the National Institute of Genetics in Mishima. In 1990, the latter was processing about 3% of all the DNA sequencing produced worldwide while the remaining 97% was held at EMBL and GenBank.

Also, there are several repositories for the biological materials that are generated by genome studies. The American Type Culture Collection (ATCC) in Rockville, Maryland maintains a variety of animal, plant, and bacterial cell lines, viral and other vectors, as well as an NIH-sponsored collection of human DNA probes and chromosome libraries. The ATCC amplifies, stores, and distributes them along with specific information to investigators. The recipients must agree to not use the material for commercial purposes nor to sell it.

The Human Genetic Mutant Cell Repository at the Coriell Institute for Medical Research in Camden, New Jersey is sponsored by the National Institute of General Medical Sciences of NIH. It contains a large collection of well-characterized human cell cultures, including material from family groups which are useful for linkage analyses.

As a means of relating to available data bases, there are two resources which link investigators to genome research projects. The "List of Molecular Biology" (LiMB) at Los Alamos National Laboratory supplies information on the means of accessing the contents of the major foreign and U.S. data bases relating to molecular biology. The "Directory of Biotechnology Information Resources" (DBIR) of the National Library of Medicine provides information on a wide range of resources relative to biotechnology.

This rather mundane listing of the principal existing data bases and repositories may give the impression that any problems relative to the storage and retrieval of information and materials generated by genome analyses have been solved. As a matter of fact, a major initiative spelled out in the DOE/NIH five-year plan for the HGP has to do precisely with a critically needed improvement of genome "informatics"—that scientific discipline that includes all of the varied aspects of information acquisition, processing, storage, distribution, analysis, and interpretation.

The massive amount and extraordinary complexity of mapping and sequencing data which will be generated by the HGP has necessitated the development of a coordinated national program so that the information and tools of analysis will be available to the widest possible range of scientists and physicians in a useful form and in a timely cost-effective fashion.

The goals of the five-year plan in this regard are to (1) develop effective software and data base design to support large-scale mapping and sequencing projects, and (2) create data base tools that provide easy access to up-to-date physical mapping, genetic mapping, chromosome mapping, and sequencing information, and allow ready comparison of the data in these several data sets.

In late 1990 it was still not even clear whether the most useful informatics system would be a single, large data base or a set of smaller networked data bases. No decision had been made on how such data bases would be constructed or even whether the existing data bases could be adapted to meet the long-term needs of the HGP! In June 1986, four years after being established, GenBank reported that it was two years behind in data entry. By 1990, it was a year behind and it took several hours to match a given sequence for all others in the data base. The flood of data—at least 100 times the amount stored by 1990—that would flow from the HGP simply could not be handled efficiently as the project began.

In an attempt to assist themselves in developing data management programs, in 1990 the DOE and NIH established a "Joint Informatics Task Force" (JITF). The group was headed by Dieter Söll of Yale University and included recognized experts in the fields of molecular biology and computer science from academia, government, and industry. Their initial efforts focused on the development of mapping and sequencing software tools and the rapid and convenient dissemination of genetic mapping and DNA sequence data.

In addition, their long-term goals included: (1) standards for connecting the many data bases being developed in individual laboratories; (2) assisting in networking among the human genome research community; and (3) planning creative interactions among computer scientists, mathematicians, and biologists by coordinating meetings, workshops, and courses.

Genome data bases are and will continue to be essential resources for a diverse user population. Biochemists, for example, can use the sequencing and protein data to create genetically engineered organisms that can produce currently scarce or unavailable medically significant human proteins and hormones. Physicians will use the genetic and sequence data to understand, diagnose, and treat human genetic disease. Evolutionary biologists need the data on relationships between sequences to trace the origins of and connections among diverse groups of living organisms.

The invaluable genome information resources supporting the HGP must be a coordinated, integrated network into which data can be conveniently entered and from which information and all its relationships with other existing information can be accessed. But as the HGP officially began its journey toward acquiring "fundamental information needed to further our basic scientific understanding of human genetics in the role of various genes in health and disease," neither the sequencing technology nor the informatics capabilities were sufficient to achieve those ends.

          *   *   *

As the details of genetic and physical maps continue to accumulate, specific genes are being located and analyzed. Prominent among them are genes which cause human disease. The isolation, cloning, and analysis of these genes and their use in the diagnosis and perhaps even the treatment of the often devastating diseases which they cause is already being made possible by the research being carried out in the name of the Human Genome Project.

8

DISEASE, DIAGNOSIS, AND THERAPY

Our chromosomes may house a total of more than 100,000 genes. Most of the instructions emanating from these DNA codes initiate and integrate a complex variety of chemical reactions characteristic of a normal, healthy organism. Genes direct the synthesis of enzymes and these in turn control the cell's metabolism, which more often than not functions normally—with some notable exceptions.

Some genes, buried within our chromosomes, may be damaged and flawed but remain active. They can cause often rare but devastating physical and mental disease. For example, 30% of the young patients admitted to pediatric hospitals in North America have diseases that can be traced directly to genetic causes. More and more we are recognizing that genetic flaws also contribute to many common disease conditions such as cancer, heart disease, and diabetes.

The urge to understand how we and other living organisms function at the cellular and molecular level has been a major impetus for scientific investigation. The enormous possibilities inherent in mapping and sequencing genomes have fueled these studies with a sense of urgency, which is further compounded by a new hope of relieving human suffering.

Even a slight genetic error can derail protein production, resulting in disease and deformity. More than 3000 inherited diseases are thought to be due to aberrations in single genes! Many more are influenced by combinations of genes. The major participants in the HGP are uniquely qualified by experience and orientation to bring particular attention to bear on those altered genes which are the agents of disease.

The Department of Energy has a congressional mandate to monitor inherited damage due to low-level exposure to radiation. The DOE Los Alamos National Laboratory has been the home of GenBank, the major U.S. DNA sequence data base, since 1983. A major portion of the research in human genetics and the breakthroughs in DNA methodology have been supported by NIH funding. The Howard Hughes Medical Institute (HHMI) has long supported biomedical research on basic genetic mechanisms and genetic disease as well as supplying funding for the Human Gene Mapping Library and the "On-Line Mendelian Inheritance in Man" data bases. HHMI also collaborates with the Center for the Study of Human Polymorphisms (CEPH) headquartered in Paris, France.

In addition, the study of the inheritance patterns of disease related to specific genes has traditionally supported the mapping of genes to their relative positions on specific chromosomes. It is not surprising then that many of the early successes flowing from the initiatives that sparked the HGP have been those that have located and characterized human disease genes.

Our search for the sites of our genes has just begun. Only about 5000 have been assigned to approximate locations on our chromosomes. However, in the 1980s and 1990s the emerging technology of mapping and sequencing—made possible first by the molecular biology revolution of the 1970s—has already produced some remarkable discoveries about the location and function of a variety of devastating genetic disorders. Diagnosis has become possible, diseased genes have been isolated, and the way to prevention, treatment, or cure can now reasonably be sought. This chapter is the story of how some of those discoveries have come about and what this means to the human condition.

GENETIC DISEASE

The history of humankind is a story of the struggle to gain control over our surroundings, particularly in so far as they impinge on our safety and comfort. The growth of agriculture, shelter, transportation, and all such various accomplishments contributing to the definition of civilization have sought to keep nature at bay and, too often destructively, to bend it to our will. Whatever control we may have gained over disease is largely a product of the twentieth century.

Idealize if you wish the "noble savage," but life for the human species has been an experience marked by almost unrelieved suffering at the hands of invisible agents. Any insight into the role of bacteria and viruses in disease is a recent phenomenon. So too has been the realization that inheritable diseases are governed by genes which are passed on from generation to generation. The effects of such disease arise from causes not from our surroundings, but from deep within our very cells.

The mid-1940s can truly be said to have ushered in the age of modern medicine. Antibiotics, first in the form of penicillin which became available only near the end of the World War II, have since been followed by an increasing number of antibacterial medications and immunizations against bacteria and viral pathogens. Humans had, for the first time, both preventive measures and effective therapeutic agents against infectious disease.

Genetic disease presents an entirely different scenario. The effects of sickle-cell anemia, adenosine deaminase (ADA) deficiency, retinoblastoma, Tay–Sachs syndrome, polycystic kidney disease, cystic fibrosis, Huntington's disease, and a host of other conditions lend themselves only to palliative measures at best. They are caused by genes whose very existence until recently were unknown. Even after the role of those genes and their molecular architecture were revealed, the genes themselves remained as remote and inaccessible as ever. Then came the miracle of molecular biology and the realization began to dawn that the gene might in fact be amenable to direct manipulation.

Is it any wonder that this possibility has captured the imagination of scientists? The HGP is a frontal assault on the genetic fate dealt to each human. The mapping and sequencing of genes is intended to lead to knowledge that will allow diagnosis, treatment, cure, and prevention of the genetic diseases that diminish the lives of so many people.

Questions may legitimately be raised about whether or not these ends are best achieved by a research effort on such a grand scale as the HGP but one would have difficulty questioning the intellectual and emotional appeal of the opportunity to gain some measure of control over our genetic inheritance. Another chapter will look at the ethical issues raised by such power over human inheritance. Here we will explain the science, what has been done and what waits in the wings.

Let's briefly review a few concepts necessary to follow the details of genetic disease research. A gene, through the intermediary messenger RNA, directs the synthesis of a chain of amino acids. This chain is the polypeptide which may, by itself or in conjunction with one or more other polypeptides, assume a complex three-dimensional configuration and become a protein. Some of these proteins act as enzymes, catalysts that drive the chemical reactions of the living cell. When we study the function of a gene we are focusing on one tiny corner of a vast network of interrelated metabolic reactions.

A defective gene is one which may no longer carry the correct code in the form of a nitrogenous base sequence for a particular polypeptide. The incorrect message may be expressed as an incorrect amino acid sequence and the protein can no longer function as a catalyst. As a result, a particular chemical reaction is blocked and as a corollary, all of the reactions that would normally have occurred as a result of that initial reaction are likewise halted. A typical case would be the situation in which the correct gene for converting the amino acid phenylalanine to tyrosine is missing. The result is phenylketonuria (PKU) which causes brain damage and diminished head size.

As mentioned a number of times, we carry two copies of most of our genes in the nucleus of each cell with the exception of the gametes, which retain only one copy after their formation by meiosis. The pairs of genes (the alleles) occur at the same site on both members of a chromosome pair, one inherited from the male and the other from the female parent. If the genes are identical, the person is homozygous for those alleles and if they differ, she or he is heterozygous.

A gene causing a defect may be either dominant or recessive, depending on the disease in question. If dominant, it can exert its effects even in the heterozygous condition; if it is recessive, the homozygous condition must be present. If the recessive disease gene is present in a heterozygous setting, that is, paired with a dominant gene, it will remain silent and unexpressed. The person heterozygous for that gene is a "carrier." Only when two recessive genes, one from each of two carriers, combines in the act of fertilization between the sperm and the egg, each containing 23 chromosomes, to reconstitute the full complement of 46 human chromosomes, can the symptoms of the disease appear.

The sex of humans is determined by the presence of two sex chromosomes. The female has two X chromosomes while the male contains one X and one Y in each cell. The X chromosomes are homologous, but the X bears many loci which are not present on the smaller Y chromosome. Defective genes on the X are therefore more apt to be expressed in the male due to the lack of a corresponding allele. They are not functional in the female unless she is homozygous recessive.

Most genetic diseases that are caused by single-gene defects are due to recessive alleles. Since two of these must occur together in the homozygous state, one can understand why marriages between two closely related people would be more apt to bring together two recessives since the gene in question would be distributed within that related group. It has been established that first cousin marriages account for about 20% of albino children and as many as 53% of children with the fatal Tay–Sachs disease. Even though the majority of the recognized recessive genetic diseases are quite rare, in combination they represent an enormous burden of human suffering.

There are several well-known disease states attributable to dominant alleles. Achondroplasia (a kind of dwarfism), Huntington's disease, and brachydactyly (very short fingers) are caused by the presence of a dominant allele. Another is hypercholesterolemia, characterized by elevated blood levels of cholesterol and resulting in heart attacks. It is considered to be the most common genetic disorder, inherited in Mendelian fashion. It affects one out of every 500 people.

Other disorders are sex-linked. Duchenne muscular dystrophy and hemophilia result from genes on the X chromosome, accounting for the fact that such conditions are very rare in females. They would need two affected X chromosomes in order to exhibit the disease state. Please note that although there is a large category of diseases traced to single-gene defects, some fatal and others with varying degrees of severity, many genetic disease conditions are due to a complexity of interacting genes.

Multifactorial complex diseases, such as atherosclerosis, or vascular disease, are prominent examples. Also, some forms of cancer require the

presence of both cancer-causing genes and defects in tumor-suppressor
genes. Problems caused by multiple genes are much more difficult to
trace and to analyze so that most of the attention has been focused on
single-gene defects which are also more amenable to treatment.

We have already introduced the concepts of mapping and sequencing in earlier chapters. Now let's look at several outstanding examples of
how such advances have been appropriated to seek out prominent disease
genes. They are also examples of "reverse genetics." This means that one
is able to find at least the approximate location of a gene or genes that
cause(s) a disease in which one has no idea of the specific biochemical
defect involved. This is in contrast to a disease such as sickle-cell
anemia, in which there is an obvious defect in the hemoglobin-carrying
red blood cells which points to a probable defect within the hemoglobin
gene. These examples of reverse genetics can be thought of as a paradigm
for what scientists can expect to accomplish through the HGP.

Let's look at the recent detective work that has contributed to our
current understanding of several major human genetic diseases. Direct
treatment of the genetic flaws underlying these conditions is not now
possible. We will conclude with a discussion of the scientific bases for the
hopes that this may be within our reach.

Cystic Fibrosis

In Chapter 1 we introduced the story of the search for the cystic
fibrosis gene. Cystic fibrosis (CF) is an inherited disease that affects the
lungs, pancreas, and sweat glands. The symptoms appear in infancy and
are characterized by chronic lung infection, abnormal pancreatic function, and a high salt content in the sweat. These are due to the fact that
there is a defect in certain pores in the membranes of cells which fails to
allow chloride to enter the cells. The result is a thick mucus which clogs
the respiratory passages in the lungs and plugs the ducts of the pancreas
and liver, interfering with breathing and digestion. Those with CF
usually succumb to respiratory infections.

CF affects 1 in every 1800 white and 1 in every 17,000 black people.
One out of 22 whites carries the recessive gene and CF is present when

there is a homozygous combination of two recessive genes. The average survival age of people with CF is 25 years.

After seven years of intensive searching, a team of Canadian and American researchers located this recessive gene. In 1985, Lap-Chee Tsui and John R. Riordan at Toronto's Hospital for Sick Children had mapped it to chromosome 7 by gene linkage analysis using RFLPs. Patterns of inheritance within hundreds of families affected by cystic fibrosis were studied. The investigators found two marker sites which were located on either side of an area on chromosome 7, as indicated by the fact that these markers were typically inherited along with the disease.

The chromosomal area flanked by the markers was isolated by a combination of human–rodent cell hybrids and restriction enzyme gene mapping, assisted by gel electrophoresis. Many pieces of DNA fragments from a flow-sorted genomic library specific to chromosome 7 were cloned. By 1988, the distance between the markers had been "reduced" to a distance of 1.5 million base pairs. There remained the formidable task of searching that long nitrogenous base sequence for the deficient gene. This was accomplished by chromosome "walking" and "jumping."

"Walking" along a chromosome is a term used to describe a technique which sometimes permits one to isolate a gene sequence when its approximate location is known. One begins with the DNA segment that contains the gene as well as an additional length of DNA containing an area that always hybridizes to a particular probe. The probe is used as a starting point to try to isolate the disease-specific gene itself. A clone is isolated from a genomic library that contains a segment of the genome corresponding to the probe. A portion of the clone farthest away from the probe hybridization site is isolated and used to rescreen the library for new clones that overlap it but are still farther away from the first probe.

This process is repeated many times and one "walks along" toward the area of the gene in steps of 20 or so kilobases. This is a slow, tedious process and can be accelerated by "jumping."

This refers to the practice of using restriction enzymes which cut the DNA infrequently and thus generate larger fragments, thereby furnishing longer probing distances. The use of PAGE and YACs allow the handling and cloning of these large fragments. A key difference between walking and jumping is that in the latter the large DNA fragments are formed into circles and the DNA from the area where the circle closes is cut out and cloned, thus bringing together DNA sequences that were originally far apart on the DNA. These cloned DNAs from the closure site make up a "jumping" library. In the case of the CF gene search, jumps of up to 100 kb were possible with this shortcut.

By January 1989 the researchers, now joined by Dr. Francis Collins of the Howard Hughes Medical Institute and the University of Michigan, had narrowed the search to a stretch of about 300,000 base pairs big enough to account for several genes. Then walking took over to move along the DNA in small increments so as not to pass over the CF gene. Several other approaches were used in these final stages. For example, all of the messenger RNA made by cells in human sweat glands was extracted and cDNAs were prepared. These were used as probes to locate a large gene extending across about 250,000 bases in a mosaic composed of 24 exons separated by noncoding introns. The gene turned out to be missing only three nitrogenous bases that coded for inserting phenyl-alanine into position 508 in a polypeptide. The cystic fibrosis gene had been found.

The news made world headlines. Hopes were raised for the possi-bility of accurate diagnostic tests for carriers and perhaps even treatment for those with the disease. However, as it turned out, 70% of the defective CF genes were missing the code for phenylalanine while 30% of the CF genes had at least one other form of the mutation not yet analyzed. As the months passed after the initial euphoria, researchers across the world found to their growing surpise and discontent that more than 40 different mutations are capable of causing CF, thus making it impossible to develop a convenient prenatal screening test which would detect all forms of the gene.

There are striking racial and geographic differences. In Denmark, for example, 90% of the CF mutations involve the loss of phenylalanine while in Israel only 30% of CF mutations involve this loss. This has slowed the development of a satisfactory prenatal screening test, which to be accurate would have to detect the vast majority of CF-causing mutations.

The multiplicity of mutations that can cause CF also complicates the problem of understanding how the gene defect causes the disease. Researchers still do not know what specific protein the gene encodes, although the most favorable hypothesis is that it is a protein dubbed CFTR, or "cystic fibrosis transmembrane conductance regulator." That protein is necessary to control the passage of chloride across cell membranes.

On September 20, 1990, newspapers carried the dramatic announcement that two research groups, using viruses as vectors, had introduced normal genes into cystic fibrosis lung cells growing in the laboratory. The genes began making the proteins that cystic fibrosis patients lack. This may lead the way in years to come to translate this into a therapy for humans, perhaps by packaging these normal genes in harmless viruses that would be inhaled in nasal spray.

Huntington's Disease

Equally tantalizing and frustrating has been the remarkable progress in the quest for the genetic cause of Huntington's disease (HD), a relatively rare disorder. Traced to the effects of a single dominant gene, the onset of this tragic disorder is insidious. There is a gradual degeneration of nerve cells in the brain which may begin as early as the age of 2 or as late as a person's 80s but usually exhibits its deadly symptoms in mid-life. The disease achieved notoriety during the 1960s when it led to the death of the beloved folk singer Woody Guthrie.

The duration of the disease can be as long as 25 years, during which time there is gradual loss of control over the voluntary muscles, first causing twitches, then large random motions followed by dementia and finally death. Tragically, people with HD maintain a social intelligence— an awareness that they can no longer control their physical faculties and are unable to communicate their needs and feelings to others.

Unlike almost all other genetic diseases, HD inexplicably has a delayed onset, becoming evident in many cases long after the affected individual has become a parent. Since a dominant gene is responsible, each child of a parent with the disease has a 50–50 chance of inheriting it. Before 1983, diagnosis of a parent after the symptoms had become unmistakable told the offspring only these odds. Since that time the presence of the gene has been detectable through an RFLP marker.

The path that led to this unique marker began long before 1983. In 1955, Americo Negrette, a physician working at a military base near Lake Maracaibo, Venezuela, documented the disease among the inhabitants of a cluster of nearby small villages. At first Dr. Negrette thought that many of the villagers whom he had often observed staggering about the streets were drunk. When it was finally explained to him that they were ill, he began taking careful histories and determined that this was, in fact, HD, or as it was then called, Huntington's "chorea," meaning "dancelike movement."

Nancy Wexler, a clinical psychologist, has both a professional and personal interest in HD. Her mother had succumbed to the disease so that Wexler and her sister were at risk. Her father, Dr. Milton Wexler, had established the Hereditary Disease Foundation dedicated to finding a cure for HD as well as to support research in other areas of inheritable diseases. Nancy Wexler and her colleagues successfully recommended that NIH initiate a study of the unique Venezuelan population.

When the research group first went to Venezuela in 1979 their intent was to search out someone who was homozygous for the gene. Once they had begun field work in earnest in 1981, however, recombinant DNA technology had expanded to the point where their emphasis switched from only classical genetic linkage studies to collecting blood samples from which to extract DNA for RFLP analysis. As it turned out, the family tree which they uncovered was far beyond their expectations. It included over 10,000 people and has proven to be a rich resource for understanding inheritance in general as well as providing a major genetic linkage reference for other diseases.

HD is a perfect example of what is known in genetics as the "founder effect." This refers to a high frequency of a gene in a population because that population began or was "founded" with a small number of people, at least one of whom carried the gene in question. Interbreeding within the initial limited population spread the gene. The Venezuelan group has been traced back seven generations to a woman whose father, a European, carried the defective gene.

There is another intensively studied populaton in southeastern

Australia where records show that least 432 Australian HD sufferers have inherited the gene of an English widow, a Miss Cundick, who took her 13 children from two marriages and emigrated to Australia in 1848.

James Gusella, Michael Conneally, and a large team of collaborators at Massachusetts General Hospital had spent a decade trying to find a gene linked to the inheritance of HD but to no avail. Almost immediately after they began to look for an RFLP marker associated with it, they succeeded. They found a hybridizing probe which they called G8 among the first dozen that they tried. This probe hybridized to an RFLP that is very close to the HD gene. The gene turned out to be located on chromosome 4 as determined by probing human–mouse hybrid cell lines. Only the cell line containing chromosome 4 hybridized with the G8 probe.

The inheritance pattern is somewhat complicated in that there are four possible variations of the RFLPs that can be found in the affected families. Each person receives two RFLP patterns, one from each of the parents. Southern hybridizations of restriction enzyme fragments from the DNA of a Venezuelan individual showing the so-called "C" pattern have the disease or will develop it later on in life. In contrast, other families in other countries may have the "A" type of RFLP pattern. There is variation here but the RFLP type remains consistent within a family grouping.

So far, scientists are within a few million bases of the gene. Unfortunately, the sequence within the area of the gene is of such a base pattern that restriction enzymes tend to cut it into many small fragments, making a detailed mapping of the region very difficult to construct. New RFLPs must be found closer to the gene and flanking it on either side. Then, once the search has been narrowed to a piece of DNA approximately 500 kb or less, chromosome jumping and walking can proceed with some reasonable chance of success.

The exact nature of the HD gene itself, unlike that of the CF gene, remains a mystery but with the RFLP markers diagnosis is possible. The child of a parent with HD now has the option to have an RFLP analysis to ascertain the presence of the deadly dominant gene. Should the person undergo the test and discover either that she or he lacks the defective gene or harbors it in every cell? If the HD gene is not there this means that none of her or his children are at risk (assuming that the other parent is negative as well). If the gene is found, the person can look forward to undergoing the same progressive loss of physical integrity that he or she has witnessed in his or her parent.

The odds are 50–50 of passing the gene on to his or her children. RFLPs, chromosome jumping, PCR, and other molecular genetics technology takes on a new air of importance when viewed by those who look to them as the only means of isolating and cloning the gene which lies waiting in their DNA like a time bomb. When the gene is isolated and its function understood, scientists hope that some form of gene therapy may be possible.

Alzheimer's Disease

The data collected from the massive Venezuelan family network has been used for studying a whole array of genetic diseases. Normal maps of gene marker locations have been made by using the Venezuelan family samples. These normal maps are then compared with the chromosome maps of other family groups exhibiting other diseases of interest, families that are often too small to be used for productive mapping.

Prominent among the genes that the Venezuelan samples have helped to map is the gene for familial Alzheimer's disease (AD). This condition presents a complex and frustrating interplay between genetic and other often undetermined factors. While genetics undoubtedly plays a role, and up to 50% of the members of some families develop Alzheimer's, this accounts for fewer than 1 of 20 who have the disease.

AD may afflict more than 10% of people aged 65 and older and nearly 50% of those 80 years and above. It is a degenerative disorder of the central nervous system characterized by impairment of memory and intellectual function often resulting in a profound mental and physical disability that may necessitate institutional care. Death usually occurs within five to ten years after the onset of symptoms. AD costs an estimated $25 billion per year in the United States alone. Of course, the cost in suffering for the patients and their families is incalculable.

No effective treatment for either preventing or arresting the progress of AD has been found. In 1987, a 22-member international research team reported tracing the genetic defect causing family-related AD to chromosome 21. Interestingly, this is the same chromosome implicated in Down's syndrome, a very common form of mental retardation. It is almost always caused by the presence of an extra chromosome 21 in each cell. People with Down's syndrome, if they live long enough, often develop AD. Again, the promise held out by finding markers linked to the AD gene is that it narrows the search for the gene itself.

An understanding of the AD defect at the molecular level might make it possible to define the biochemical pathways involved in the initiation and progress of the chemical and neuropathological features of the disease. Brain disorders are very difficult to treat. Most drugs, though they may circulate freely in the blood, cannot leave the blood vessels and enter brain tissue. Neurons, the cell type that makes up most of the brain and nerves, cannot be removed and treated without causing serious damage.

However, experiments with animals indicate that it may be possible to implant genetically altered fibroblasts (connective tissue cells) into the brain, where they stimulate release of a nerve growth factor in the kind of neurons whose malfunction is associated with memory loss in Alzheimer's disease. This may prove to be a useful gene delivery system when causative genes are eventually isolated.

Clues may also be found as to how environmental factors affect nongenetic AD. Meanwhile, as the gene hunt continues, the National Institute on Aging estimates that as many as 14 million Americans will have Alzheimer's disease by the middle of the next century.

Neurofibromatosis

The Venezuelan family studies have contributed as well to the pursuit of the neurofibromatosis (NF) gene. NF, known earlier by the equally polysyllabic designation of von Recklinghausen's disease, is probably best known to the general public as the presumed cause of the grotesque disfigurement of John Merrick, the late-nineteenth century "elephant man." Merrick, the subject of a recent popular movie and play, was an exceptional example of a disease which is actually one of the most prevalent of genetic diseases, affecting 1 in 4000 people. Actually, as it turned out, Merrick probably suffered from another disorder with similar symptoms, the rare Proteus syndrome.

NF is typically characterized by light brown spots and skin lumps caused by underlying nerve tumors which in one third of the patients often causes loss of hearing and sight and other serious neurological difficulties. There is no treatment possible other than surgery to remove the tumors which frequently return. In May 1987, two groups, one at the University at Utah and the other at Massachusetts General Hospital, located the gene, a dominant allele, on chromosome 17.

As soon as the home of the gene had been discovered, numerous investigators joined their efforts in a consortium sponsored by the National Neurofibromatosis Foundation, exchanging cell lines and DNA markers to fix its position. By early 1988, the location was reduced to a 3 million base stretch, a formidable maze of DNA that might have required years of analysis were it not for two NF patients who turned out to have distinctive landmarks within that region. In one, chromosome 17 had broken and exchanged a piece with chromosome 1; in the other there had been an exchange between chromosome 17 and chromosome 22. The working assumption was made that these two disruptions were within the NF gene and had thus caused the disease.

Two groups, one led by Francis Collins of CF gene fame and the other by Raymond White at the University of Utah, both funded by the Howard Hughes Medical Institute, began to collaborate closely in the investigation. They scoured the area around the chromosome breakage points, which were about 60 kb apart, looking for an expressed gene. To their surprise they found several. During the effort to distinguish one from the other, Collins' group found a person with NF whose DNA had an extra 500-base segment in the middle of one of the candidate genes. The patient's parents did not have the insert.

The gene turned out to be an intriguing entity, unlike any other human gene discovered up until then. It was between 500 and 2000 kb in length and there were at least three other genes embedded within it. Another example of such a "nested" gene is one buried within the factor VIII hemophilia gene on the X chromosome. In both cases what was so suprising, in addition to the demonstration that genes could be embedded in others, was that the embedded genes were oriented in the opposite direction. Their nitrogenous base code would have to be read, as it were, from left to right instead of right to left like all other known genes. Findings like this show that genomes may be much more complex than previously thought.

By the time the gene was located, the two groups of Collins and White had gone their separate ways and both, amazingly, came to the same conclusions at almost the same time. Such internecine rivalries are common in science. They are usually based on a disagreement, as in this case, stemming from the question of which approach will be the most productive. Rather than engendering hostility, the creative tension induced by such a "race" is often fruitful, stimulating each group to prove itself correct in the competition.

As we have pointed out, the determination of the exact location of the gene should help with diagnosis, which can be difficult in children under the age of 5. An improved prenatal test should be possible as well. The problem with such a large gene is that almost every family that has the disease has a slightly different version of the gene. Even so, a test which detects the majority of the mutations would be very useful.

It looks as if the gene may belong to the recently discovered class of "tumor suppressive" genes. This means that the normal gene acts to inhibit new tumor development and certain mutations serve to inactivate the gene so that it can no longer play its inhibitory role.

Thus, the NF gene may be a factor in other tumors as well. This may explain the variable manifestations of the gene. Perhaps two mutations are needed to bring on the disease as has been found to be the case with retinoblastoma, a rare eye cancer. Further study of the NF gene may uncover information on the complex factors that affect stimulation and inhibition of cell growth.

Cancer

The role of genetics in cancer has become much better understood since 1975. That year marked the astonishing Nobel-prize-winning dis-

covery by J. Michael Bishop and Harold E. Varmies of the University of
California at San Francisco that human cells harbor genes which can turn
against their host and cause cancer. Instead of seeing cancer as an outside
intruder, scientists now understand it as disease brought about by genes
often influenced by external stimuli.

A gene which normally plays a useful role in cells, such as
controlling growth, may become damaged from a wide variety of
causes—by a virus, a chemical, radiation, or some other external agent.
It becomes an "oncogene" whose code has become flawed, turning it
into a potential killer.

This discovery and the subsequent worldwide study of its implications have turned up a frustratingly complicated array of oncogenes. For
example, scientists analyzing tumors from the breast, colon, bladder, and
lungs have found more than 50 types of oncogenes.

In 1982, Robert Weinberg established that an oncogene that caused
bladder cancer in humans was almost identical to a viral oncogene that
caused tumors in rats. This discovery of the so-called "*ras*" gene helped
to unify the study of oncogenes. Cancer-causing retroviruses apparently
first pick up the oncogene in its messenger RNA form during the infection
of a cell. The viruses then incorporate it into their own RNA. When the
virus later infects other cells and inserts its RNA inside it, the resultant
"stolen" gene code causes the cell to grow out of control and develop into
a tumor.

This discovery focused scientists on the problem of how these genes
instigate such a transformation. For example, studies of the rare child-
hood cancer retinoblastoma have shown that it is not caused by an
oncogene that turns on growth but by the lack of genes that normally
switch off growth. The consensus now is that most cancers are caused by
a series of molecular accidents—changes in normal genes (the "proto-
oncogenes") that then turn into oncogenes and disrupt the normal
mechanisms of growth and development. Some of these changes may be
inherited while others are acquired from exposure to external agents,
"carcinogens" such as chemicals or radiation.

A study in 1989 found that tumors containing multiple copies of an
oncogene known as *HER*-2/*neu* may be indicative of a faster growing
form of the disease. This may lead the way to using gene probes to assess

patients' prospects. Whatever form of cancer one examines, it is obvious that a major gap in our understanding of cancer is how the function of a specific oncogene is related to the progressive events that culminate in a life-threatening tumor.

As we have pointed out earlier, the appeal made by the internationally recognized Renato Dulbecco in March 1986 in support of sequencing the entire human genome—thus supplying probes for all the genes—was based on the conviction that such knowledge would be the major turning point in cancer research. This turned out to be a major impetus in generating the birth of the HGP.

Duchenne Muscular Dystrophy

The most common form of muscular dystrophy, Duchenne muscular dystrophy (DMD), is another devastating genetic disease that affects as many as 1 out of every 3500 male infants. It first exhibits symptoms of muscle weakness between the ages of 3 to 7 and thereafter there is progressive muscle degeneration. Most of these children die in their late teens or early 20s when the chest muscles needed for breathing or the heart muscle finally give out.

The fact that the gene or genes responsible must be on the X chromosome has long been evident because of the inheritance pattern. Only very rarely does a female inherit the disease. The study of 12 young women with DMD showed that they all had an X chromosome broken in about the same place—a band called Xp21 toward one end of the X chromosome. That indicated that probably the break had occurred somewhere within the DMD gene, inactivating it and thereby causing the disease.

In 1986, Louis Kunkel, a geneticist at Harvard Medical School, and his colleagues succeeded in isolating and cloning the DMD gene. It is another enormous gene, spanning 1 to 2 million bases and containing at least 60 exons. It codes for a correspondingly large protein called "dystrophin," which is about ten times the size of an average polypeptide. The scientific collaboration that led all the way to dystrophin is an excellent example of international cooperation. One scientific paper alone related to the project listed 77 authors from 24 research institutions in 8 countries. Probes, clones, and patient samples were freely exchanged, all of which ultimately led researchers to their quarry.

Researchers hope to develop procedures to inject genes coding for dystrophin, a structural component of normal muscle, directly into muscles. Some experiments have shown that gene injections into animal muscle have stimulated production of protein by muscle cells for several months.

GENETIC DIAGNOSIS AND THERAPY

Numerous other examples could be cited of disease genes that have been mapped to specific chromosomes. Let us assume that many such genes have been located and that someday they, like the several that we have explained in some detail, will have been isolated and cloned. What are the implications of having specific genes in our possession?

We already have seen that even an RFLP marker for a gene is a powerful aid in the confirmation of the presence of that gene at any stage of development from prenatal to adulthood. The power of this diagnostic capability is just beginning to be felt in such tragic diseases as Huntington's. With the advances that will surely flow from the HGP, the list of diagnosable disorders through genetic analysis will grow rapidly.

Such genetic diagnosis may determine the presence or absence of a particular gene. If the report is negative, those involved are relieved of an enormous burden of concern. If a positive finding confirms that the gene is present, what then?

If the finding is at the prenatal stage, the information is added to the complex of medical and ethical bases on which an abortion decision is to be made. Such decisions often already include fetal chemical and cytological tests which can indicate the presence or absence of numerous medical problems. RFLP tests will soon add very many more disease states to this list.

When a genetic disease is diagnosed after birth, what then? Traditionally, treatment to relieve the symptoms has been all that was possible.

Now, many of the molecular biology techniques which we have introduced in these chapters are being utilized in an attempt to gain some measure of control over our genomes. The varied procedures that attempt to do this are referred to as "gene therapy."

No other area in molecular genetics is as rife with promise and controversy as gene therapy. We will treat its social and ethical implications in later chapters. Here we will look at its science, the biological principles of genetic manipulation which tries to alter our genetic inheritance.

Consider the explicit and implicit problems. Our genes are part of the chromosomes which function within the nucleus of each cell. Every defective gene is therefore inside each diploid somatic (nonreproductive) cell and distributed at random in the haploid gametes. The aim of gene therapy is to replace or supplement the defective genetic information with normal, functional genes. How could we possibly get at those undesirable genes, hidden as they are inside the trillions of cells that constitute the human body?

The actual physical removal and replacement of genes in the body's cells is not possible. However, ample precedent exists for the introduction of normal genes into cells where they become part of the functional genome of the cell without necessitating the removal or repair of a resident nonfunctional gene.

This incorporation of foreign DNA into bacteria, which we described in the gene cloning process as "transformation," in other kinds of cells is known as "transfection." DNA can be introduced into cells by a variety of methods including direct uptake in the presence of chemicals such as calcium phosphate, exposure of cells to rapid pulses of high-voltage current (electroporation), and direct injection of the DNA into cells through ultrathin glass needles (microinjection).

The problem is not completely one of getting DNA into the genome of cells in the laboratory. One major problem is that transfection is random. This means that there is at present no way to insert the DNA into a genome in a position where it is sure not to interfere with the normal functioning of that genome. A DNA segment that becomes inserted into a proto-oncogene might trigger a cancer or the interference of such DNA with a promoter sequence could destroy the function of a healthy gene. In addition, how does one get the DNA into cells within the body where it can function to overcome the presence of the deleterious gene?

Even if the gene does enter the cell and integrates safely in the genome, this still does not mean that the introduced gene will function properly. It also needs the correct DNA sequence to "turn on" its function of coding for a polypeptide. The problems seem insurmountable—yet scientists have devised gene therapies for several human genetic diseases and await final approval for clinical trials.

The first tests leading to gene therapy were done in May 1989. At the National Institutes of Health Clinical Center a cancer patient with advanced melanoma, a dangerous skin cancer, made scientific history as he was given an infusion of his own white blood cells containing a foreign gene. The gene was one for resistance to the antibiotic neomycin and was used, not as a therapy, but to track the movement of the white blood cells in the patient's body. Technically this is considered "gene transfer" since no therapeutic gene was introduced. The tests proved that genes could, in fact, be introduced into the body and function there. The milestone study was a collaboration between Steven A. Rosenberg of the National Cancer Institute and W. French Anderson and R. Michael Blaese of the Heart Institute.

The candidate for the first human gene therapy trial was the inherited immune disorder adenosine deaminase (ADA) deficiency. The children with this genetic disease lack the enzyme that normally helps the body to break down toxic chemicals building up in certain types of white blood cells, the T-lymphocytes. The defect destroys the body's immune system and the children have no defense against infection. They succumb quickly unless kept in a sterile environment. In July 1990, for the first time in history a federal advisory board approved proposals to treat volunteers with genetically altered cells.

On September 14, 1990, again at the National Institutes of Health, a 4-year-old girl received an injection of her own white blood cells which contained normal ADA genes. The cells had first been removed from her bloodstream and the normal genes put into them by harmless virus vectors. By the time the sixth treatment had been administered in April 1991, Dr. Blaese announced that "I'm delighted at the way things are going . . . the patient's immune system seems to be improving."

The Recombinant DNA Advisory Committee (RAC), first created after the Asilomar Conference in 1975, is a panel of scientists, ethicians, and others charged with advising the NIH on genetic engineering. In addition to approving the clinical trials for ADA treatments the committee also approved a request by Steven A. Rosenberg for permission to inject gene-altered white blood cells into 50 people with advanced melanoma. The gene transfer experiments had been successful and in this case the gene would be a gene for "tumor necrosis factor" which assists in tumor destruction.

Both of these proposals are excellent examples of the problems typically involved in gene therapy and the ingenious methodologies used to surmount these difficulties. The first case, that of ADA deficiency, has several features that facilitate genetic treatment. The disease is caused by a single defective gene that makes a well-defined protein product. Also, the normal gene for ADA has been cloned. Most importantly perhaps is the fact that the gene can be easily inserted into white blood cells removed from the bone marrow of the affected person. The cells are then returned after transfection to the same person with the hope that the cells will produce the necessary enzyme.

Two aspects of this protocol are highly significant in the current approach to gene therapy. One is the use of bone marrow cells. If only mature body cells are genetically altered and then introduced into a patient, the newly modified genome would soon be lost when the cells eventually died. Bone marrow, however, is a reservoir of immature cells which constantly divide and mature into both red blood cells and certain forms of white blood cells. The marrow resides in the marrow cavities, chambers within the bone tissue. The new blood cells are released into the blood while the immature cells ("stem" cells) are constantly replaced by cell division of precursors.

White and red blood cells are constantly replaced. Red blood cells typically last about 120 days while white blood cells often last no more than a few hours. As a result, genes introduced into the genome of the proliferating stem cells will be copied and sent out within the blood cells. In theory, this would mean that the bone marrow could serve as a permanent source of blood cells carrying the inserted gene.

Bone marrow can easily be removed, treated, and replaced in the bone marrow cavities of the patient. Bone marrow transplants are routine, for example, in a case where cancerous blood-forming cells in a leukemia patient's marrow are replaced with cells from a healthy compatible donor. The human ADA gene has already been cloned successfully in bone marrow cells of mice.

In order to get the normal gene into the stem cells, retroviruses have been utilized as efficient vectors. As part of their natural life cycle, the retroviruses, some of which cause AIDS and various forms of cancer, insert a DNA copy of their RNA randomly into the chromosomes of an infected cell. For example, Richard Mulligan and his colleagues at the Massachusetts Institute of Technology placed a human globin gene into the genetic material of a retrovirus, and infected bone marrow from a mouse with the virus. When the marrow was returned to the mouse, its new red blood cells contained significant amounts of human globin protein.

The retroviruses offer several advantages over other means of transfection which usually result in gene insertion in 1% or less of the cells. With retroviruses, up to 100% of the cells can be infected and express the gene. Although we tend to think of viruses as harmful, retroviruses can be modified to render them nondestructive.

In the case of the melanoma therapy, a second approach is used. Lymphocytes isolated from a patient's tumor are often found to be specifically genetically programmed to kill that patient's cancer cells. These cells can be grown in a laboratory and returned at will to the patients bloodstream where they circulate and end up back at the tumor. This makes such cells an attractive vehicle for delivering therapeutic agents to the tumor site.

As mentioned before, Steven Rosenberg had used a gene that can be traced to see if the defense system could be transfected as a prelude to introducing genes whose products would be therapeutic for the cancer. A gene that confers resistance to the antibiotic neomycin was inserted into tumor-associated lymphocytes and these were injected into the patient from which they had been isolated.

The fate of these "tumor-infiltrating lymphocytes" (TILs) was followed by tumor biopsies and blood samples, and the cells were tested for neomycin resistance to see if the gene was functioning as planned. Rosenberg and his colleagues reported that the neomycin-resistance gene had been incorporated into 5% of the TILs. Because of the large number of lymphocytes, this is considered a very positive result.

Both of these novel approaches are the first to be attempted on humans. Waiting in the wings are a number of other methodologies, any of which might soon prove to be of immense value. These include injection of pure RNA or DNA directly into skeletal muscle, first reported in March of 1990, or the use of endothelial cells that line blood vessels as a vector for introducing normal genes into patients' tissues. In June 1990, James Wilson, working in Richard Mulligan's laboratory at the White-head Institute, published studies showing that such engineered cells had been successfully implanted in dogs.

Still in the planning stages are such approaches as the use of fibroblasts, connective tissue cells that are easily grown in the laboratory. Hereditary emphysema caused by alpha-1 antitrypsin (AAT) deficiency might be cured by using fibroblasts genetically modified by inserting human AAT by means of a retrovirus into fibroblasts. In experiments with mice, AAT was detected in the lungs one month after injection of treated fibroblasts.

If gene therapy is to become widespread, cells other than marrow cells or fibroblasts must be manipulated. There are promising reports that the genome of hepatocytes (liver cells) have been recipients of a gene used to make a receptor on the surface of liver cells needed for normal cholesterol metabolism. Lack of the gene leads to severe elevation of cholesterol levels and premature heart disease. The treated cells were successfully reintroduced into animals by injection.

Regardless of the methods, there is a clear distinction between gene therapy aimed at the nonreproductive (somatic) cells of the body and genetic manipulation involving the sex cells. The whole area of gene technology is fraught with controversy and much of it centers around the possibility of altering the genome of gametes. To do so would be to introduce new genetic material into a cell that could, through fertiliza-tion, pass its genome onto an entire human organism.

The introduced genetic material would then be "immortalized" in the sense that it could be passed on to the descendants of the original individual. This is in marked contrast to genetic changes in somatic cells which can go no further than the treated individual. The addition of new genes to a sperm or egg cell or even the cells of young embryos would not technically be gene therapy. It has been called "gene enhancement" or "germ-line gene therapy." The word "germ" comes from the Latin meaning "sprout." These are the cells from which all other cells in the organism will develop. The introduction of such "desirable" genes which would be passed on to all of the cells of the body as it developed is clearly different from procedures designed to correct existing genetic defects in one individual. This would constitute the deliberate addition of genes to an individual genome, not as a treatment, but in order to incorporate whatever genes one might decide were advantageous.

In other words, prevention of diseases caused by single-gene defects could possibly be carried out by inserting a normal copy of the gene in the fertilized egg (the zygote). This assumes, of course, that the fertilization process would be carried out in the laboratory before inserting the tiny embryo, developing from the egg, into the uterus. However, instead of trying to insert genes, it would be much simpler to discard affected zygotes and implant only embryos with a normal copy of the gene obtained through fertilization.

So germ-line gene therapy is considered mainly as a future means of introducing genes to enhance characteristics rather than as a curative. Perhaps, when the genes are available, they might be placed into the germ-line to make people more resistant to disease—or taller and more intelligent. With this, of course, we enter the controversies of eugenics, which we will soon discuss.

While some scientists puzzle over the nuances of getting genes into cells that will remain in the body and produce necessary levels of normal gene products, others are busy approaching the problem of gene treatment from a different perspective. They are developing "anti-sense" drugs.

These take advantage of the fact that each gene in the DNA double helix, as we have pointed out, carries a code which is translated into a single-stranded molecule of messenger RNA. This travels out of the nucleus and goes to the ribosomes where it serves as a pattern for production of a specific protein. This messenger RNA molecule is called the "sense" strand. An "anti-sense" drug is a laboratory-synthesized mirror image of the "sense" strand which will bind to it by a joining together of the nitrogenous bases, thus blocking protein production.

Another similar approach uses molecules that bind directly to the DNA double helix itself and prevent the production of the messenger in the first place. As more genes are isolated and sequenced, the synthesis of blocking molecules for DNA and RNA will be facilitated. Both of these kinds of pharmaceuticals are under development at several venture capital start-up companies and could begin appearing on the market by the mid-1990s.

The future will undoubtedly bring even more possibilities to enable scientists to insert, inhibit, or enhance genes at the level of a single cell or the entire organism. As more and more genes are located and isolated, increasing control over our genetic fate will emerge.

*   *   *

The genes have long been out of the bottle that Johann Meischer had placed on his laboratory shelf in 1899. Many have become experimental entities which one can analyze, synthesize, and utilize in an extraordinary exercise of control over the mechanics of living systems.

Genetic engineering is neither as difficult as we once thought it might be nor as simple as one might be led to think from the generalities of newspaper and magazine accounts of the latest advances. Despite the remarkable accomplishments of the past, the era of molecular genetics has only just begun.

Will the dawning "age of gene therapy" be an age of reason or one of bitter dispute? The HGP has already provoked many legitimate questions about a spectrum of issues ranging from controversies over how the project can most efficiently be carried out to whether or not it ought to proceed at all. Unprecedented cooperation among scientists vies with fierce competition, while all the while the leaders of the HGP remain confident of its ultimate success.

Having reviewed the science of the HGP, we need now to perceive it in terms of its context within society. When society and science meet, often a turbulent uproar follows.

9

THE PLAN: PROMISES AND PROBLEMS

The rhetoric soars in the accounts of the genesis of the HGP. Charles DeLisi, the former director of the Office of Health and Environmental Research (OHER), in a 1988 article in *American Scientist* speaks of the compelling justification as a quest that "has been an integral part of our intellectual heritage for centuries. . . . It recalls one of the three great precepts chiseled on the temple at Delphi and echoed two millennia later in Alexander Pope's *Essay on Man*: 'Know then thyself, presume not God to scan; a proper study of mankind is man. . . . the glory jest and riddle of the world.' " However, DeLisi adds that "the most frequently heard justification for the genome project are its promise of medical advances and increased economic competitiveness."

These three motivations, medical, economic, and philosophical, might seem to be strange bedfellows. Was the intent to decipher the human genome on such a grand scale predominantly an exciting intellectual exercise, a key to control over human disease, or a means of obtaining information which would be to our corporate and national economic interests?

Certainly this formative period appears as a mosaic that includes all of these elements. Undeniably, the concept of a concerted effort to analyze the human genome stirred the imaginations of those scientists who saw it as an opportunity to fulfill within their lifetime what had been a long-term goal.

But what began as a grandiose inspiration to sequence the entire human genome attracted enthusiastic, powerful supporters and equally vocal but less influential critics. As the plans, quickly expanded and as quickly modified, were subsumed under the Department of Energy and the National Institutes of Health, some initial skeptics became believers; but an undercurrent of concern began to grow. We need to show how these shadows, cast across the bright future promised by the advocates of the HGP, formed in their historical context. In the succeeding chapters we will examine the dangers, some very real and some imagined, of this revolution in the science of human genetics.

James Watson had entered the University of Chicago as an undergraduate while the Manhattan Project accelerated toward its awesome conclusion. The deadly results of that secret undertaking became known to the world at large on August 6, 1944 when the United States dropped an atomic bomb near the center of Hiroshima, Japan. The explosion killed over 71,000 people. Many died over the following years due to the insidious effects of radiation from that blast.

Forty years later, in March 1984, a scientific conference was held in the now rebuilt Hiroshima. The Japanese had dedicated the postwar city to peace. The ruins of the Institute of Industrial Development, with its dome warped by the heat of the blast, were left as a symbol of the terrible destruction. A special hospital had been built to treat people suffering from exposure to radiation, and scientists there carried on research into its effects on the bomb's survivors and their children. At the conference the participants stressed the need to use molecular DNA analytical tools in order to be able to detect directly mutations which could be inherited.

Interest in the issues raised at the conference led to another on the same subject nine months later. This time the discussions were sponsored by the United States Department of Energy (DOE) and the International Commission for Protection Against Environmental Mutagens and Carcinogens. Nineteen scientists, all leading experts in molecular biology, met in the snowy mountains of Alta, Utah in December 1984. Despite the advances that had been made over the previous few years in the technology of DNA analysis, the scientists concluded that the available methodology was still insufficient to detect mutations, estimated at approximately 30 mutations per individual genome per generation. Only a massive effort specifically designed to improve the technology by orders of magnitude would suffice. The ideas and interactions generated by the assembled researchers, many of whom had not previously met, would ultimately coalesce into the Human Genome Project.

Mortimer Mendelsohn noted, in an internal report to DOE: "A remarkable atmosphere of cooperation and mutual creativity pervaded the meeting. Excitement was infectious and ideas flowed rapidly from every direction . . . with many ideas surviving to the end." On his return to Washington from Alta, Michael Gough began work on a report of the meeting for the Office of Technology Assessment (OTA). The report had been requested by Congress, which had anticipated that controversies over Agent Orange exposure, radiation during tests in the 1950s, and exposure to mutagenic chemicals might end up in legal action against the United States government. In such an event, documented opinion on the feasibility of detecting mutations would be necessary.

Charles DeLisi read an early draft of this work of Gough and others which appeared in 1986 as "Technologies for Detecting Heritable Mutations in Human Beings." Robert Mullen Cook-Deegan, writing in the 1989–1990 HGP report published in 1990, says that DeLisi "while reading it first had the idea for a dedicated HGP." As evidence he cites DeLisi's 1988 paper in the September/October *American Scientist*.

In that paper DeLisi pointed out that proposals to sequence the human genome dated at least to 1985 at a workshop on the topic organized by Robert Sinsheimer of the University of Southern California. In October of that same year DeLisi read the draft of the OTA report and called it "the initial stimulus" leading to the Santa Fe workshop. This was an international gathering of 50 participants sponsored by the DOE which convened in March 1986.

The DOE had already established a National Gene Library Project based jointly at the Los Alamos and Lawrence Livermore laboratories. The library contained fragments of human DNA, chromosome by chromosome, made freely available to scientists. The idea of sequencing the entire human genome began to appear to DOE as a natural spin-off from the library project.

Discussion, therefore, at Santa Fe revolved around how the sequencing could be achieved, not whether it should be done at all. The participants immediately recognized that the organization of such a project would be as important as the actual technology involved. Nobel laureate Walter Gilbert of Harvard University, who along with Alan Maxam was famous for the development of the first method for sequencing DNA, proposed the establishment of a human genome institute devoted to large-scale sequencing. He suggested that initial efforts be devoted to sequencing known genes in regions of importance.

Most, however, felt that although some form of central control was needed, the work probably should be distributed to laboratories across the nation and perhaps even internationally. This would stimulate a wide range of creative solutions to the obvious need for major improvements in sequencing technology.

Linked to the technology would be ways to handle the vast amount of data that would be generated from such a project. Genbank, the United States national data base at Los Alamos National Laboratory, was already swamped with sequence information on just 6 million bases. How could it handle an expected 1000 times that much data?

Molecular biology had never been a major component of DOE programs. DeLisi wanted to change that. The Santa Fe meeting exceeded his expectations, culminating in glowing terms with his conclusion that "the objective was meritorious, obtainable and would be an outstanding achievement in modern biology." These were basically the same conclusions reached at the earlier Santa Cruz meeting. According to DeLisi, the excitement that was generated at Santa Fe "was reminiscent of those rare moments in the early phase of major new adventures, such as the Manhattan Project at Los Alamos or exploration of outer space that capture the collective imagination of a community."

A "Science Writers Workshop on Biotechnology and the Human Genome: Innovations and Impacts" was held at the Brookhaven National Laboratory on September 14–16, 1987. Sponsored by the Office of Health and Environmental Research of the DOE, it was a forum in which science writers, reporters, and other interested persons could learn about the "scope and direction of the human genome initiative and its supporting technologies."

The first speaker was Jack B. McConnell, Corporate Director of Advanced Technology for Johnson and Johnson, the pharmaceutical company. He stressed the urgency with getting on with the task, considering that the "implications for clinical medicine of knowing the sequence of the human genome are absolutely staggering." Pointing out that there is no other country in the world with such a vigorous research and development system, he went on to stress the importance of mapping and sequencing the entire human genome. He stated, "If we expect the U.S. to maintain its predominant position in the health care field and the pharmaceutical industry then we have to fully support this opportunity . . . the first group or institution to achieve access to the data contained in the human genome will be in a position to dominate the biotechnology and pharmaceutical industries for decades." Speaking against the idea of making this an international effort, he warned that "Each country might like to reserve for itself those thing which have economic value." The lines chiseled into the temple at Delphi ("Know Thyself") and the bottom line were not so far apart after all.

A more prosaic account was offered by Roger Lewin in *New Scientist*. According to Lewin, "The idea for the project came originally out of a multimillion dollar program to build the world's largest optical telescope." He was referring to a $36 million gift received by the University of California in 1984 toward the construction of a 10-meter telescope. The project was managed by Robert Sinsheimer, the Chancellor of the Santa Cruz campus and a molecular biologist. The University was required to return the funds "through a complex series of events" and Sinsheimer recalled that "a confluence of ideas then emerged as the thought that this money might instead be used to launch an institute to sequence the human genome at Santa Cruz."

In addition to participating in the effort to raise $80 million for the telescope, Sinsheimer was also part of a group trying to bring the superconducting supercollider to California. It occurred to him that perhaps "Scientific opportunities in biology were being overlooked simply because we were not thinking on an adequate scale." At the Santa Cruz meeting of molecular biologists the mood of the participants was said to oscillate between extreme skepticism and actual confidence in the feasibility of such a program. Although the plans of the institute were

never realized, according to Lewin, from this point on the drive toward a
human genome project "was essentially unstoppable."

In July 1990 in an article written by Bernard Davis of the Department
of Microbiology and Molecular Genetics at Harvard Medical
School and endorsed by 22 members of the faculty of the author's
department an even harsher view was proffered. In Davis' words the
"Human Genome Program . . . was advanced by a politically astute
administrator in the DOE convinced that the powerful tools of molecular
biology made it appropriate to introduce centrally administered 'big
science' into biomedical research. The idea quickly developed strong
political appeal." Davis goes on to suggest the need to reevaluate the
entire project.

Shortly thereafter, Martin Rechsteiner, professor and co-chair of the
Department of Biochemistry at the University of Utah, wrote an essay
which appeared in *New Scientist*. It was a blistering attack entitled "The
Folly of the Human Genome Project." His principal criticism was that
the project is "a costly, inappropriate and unwise allocation of precious
research funds," labeling it as an "engineering project" from which little
economic benefits would flow to the United States.

What had happened in the few years from the heady atmosphere of
Alta where the "excitement was infectious" or from the Santa Fe meeting
where "enthusiasm reigned?"

Certainly, many of the biologists who gathered on May 28, 1986 at
the Cold Spring Harbor Summer Symposium on the "Molecular Biology
of *Homo sapiens*" had not even known of the genome initiative discussed
at the Santa Fe meeting three months earlier. If laboratories are as Louis
Pasteur once said "The temples of the future," then Cold Spring Harbor
is surely a shrine. The mix of older and modern buildings nestled at the
head of a tranquil harbor halfway out on the north shore of Long Island,
New York, Cold Spring Harbor is the result of the merger of two
institutions. The original Biological Laboratory founded in 1890 by the
Brooklyn Institute joined in 1962 with a field station established several
years later by the Carnegie Institution.

When the 40-year-old James Watson took over the laboratory in
1968, it was in deep financial trouble. The "phage group" which had

heralded the dawn of molecular genetics in the 1940s was winding down and the trustees were thinking seriously of actually closing the laboratory. By 1990, through the creative energy of Watson, the laboratory had an endowment of $45 million and was considered, as it still is, one of the most exciting places in the world to do molecular biology. In fact, publications by Cold Spring Harbor scientists are cited more than papers coming from any other institution, according to Science Citation Index.

It has become a mecca for brilliant young molecular biologists where they can dedicate themselves to science, free of the burden of teaching or administration. According to Watson, "We rescued it [the laboratory] by doing good science." The science included work leading to the discovery in the early 1980s of the malfunctioning genes at the root of cancer.

David Smith described to the biological scientists assembled at the 1986 symposium the "near unanimous enthusiasm" of the Santa Fe workshop. He related how high-level DOE officials were encouraged to proceed. Near-term plans included establishing a scientific advisory committee to steer future decisions and the funding of proposals at the cost of a few million dollars over the next three years. Smith went on to describe three major areas of concern: the importance of improving sequencing technology, the development of a physical map for the human genome, and innovations in the area of data handling.

The meeting had been billed as a conference on the molecular biology of *Homo sapiens*, but what began as a report on the state of the art in the molecular biology of genetic disease and evolution quickly became an impromptu forum on the issue of these grandiose DOE plans. Ironically, one of the ultimate aims of molecular biology, the analysis of the complete sequence of the human genetic blueprint, was about to begin on someone else's turf.

True, the DOE had a long history of research on human mutations, DNA damage, and DNA repair. Also, they undoubtedly had experience in directing large-scale long-term interdisciplinary projects. But DOE had never had a major involvement in molecular biology research and had few senior administrators familiar with the world of genetics. Its leaders were invariably physicists who were not used to placing biology high on their list of priorities. There developed, as Roger Lewin wrote in *Science*, a "palpable unease" over the project. The symposium became a micro-cosm of the debate that would soon spill over into the scientific and popular press, where it has raged ever since.

Not everyone had come to the symposium unprepared for the issue. Sir Walter Bodmer, Director of Research at the Imperial Cancer Research Fund in London, U.K., announced in his opening remarks after summa-rizing genetics since 1964 that "establishing the human genome sequence is certainly a major challenge that must be taken up worldwide. It is probably the most important essentially technological project of its kind that can now be identified in terms of its potential contribution to human welfare."

Several other senior scientists, including James Watson and Walter Gilbert, joined in support of the idea that it was time to start the project. However, each had his own idea of who ought to do it. Gilbert preferred to leave the project to DOE stating that "We don't want NIH or NSF (National Science Foundation) running this because if they did there would be a greater likelihood that their funds for other research would be cut back." Watson, in contrast, was of the opinion that the "safe" course would be for NIH to take part, provided that special funds would be appropriated by Congress over and above the rest of the NIH monies.

Biochemist Paul Berg of Stanford University, a Nobel laureate, tried to get the participants to put the question of money aside and focus on the value of a genome sequencing project. Berg described his position as one of "qualified strong support" adding "is it worth the cost not in terms of dollars but in terms of its impact on the rest of biological science?" Despite the advice, many of the younger scientists reacted as Watson put it, with "downright hostility." They felt that a megabillion dollar project would inevitably divert money away from single investigator-initiated research grants from which flowed the livelihood for most of them and thereby retard the pace of high-quality biological and medical research.

As the controversy swirled about the halls of the week-long meeting on the otherwise placid shores of Long Island Sound, one could not say that a consensus had developed. Nevertheless, a change in emphasis had evolved that would prove to dominate increasingly the evolution of genome analysis. Maxine Singer of the National Cancer Institute had insisted that sequencing alone made little sense—more useful information would be gained if sequencing went hand in hand with other lines of inquiry, most notably genetics and biochemistry, the natural turf of scientists at NIH. "We wouldn't know if it was worth doing as a project until we've done it," she said, "but we do know when we do sequencing and biochemistry together we really learn a lot."

Other prominent researchers echoed her point. "In one sense the sequence is trivial" said David Botstein. "What we really want is a physical map of the genome. . . . The nucleotide [base] sequence is only the bare beginning. It's as if we were a primitive tribe that collected all the papers of Shakespeare on a beach and tried to put them in order. It is *Hamlet*, but we don't even know it because we can't speak English."

Walter Bodmer, while championing the goal of sequencing as achievable and economically worthwhile, nevertheless had stressed in his opening remarks that the first challenge would be to map all of the functional interesting gene clusters and obtain their precise order before "eventually determining the complete nucleotide sequence . . . gene mapping is absolutely fundamental for the application of molecular genetics to the human species."

It had become evident to many of the participants that the DOE project was not about to be derailed. Plans ought to be discussed for a parallel effort by biologists which would begin with genome mapping.

Another force was operative as well that week in June 1986, as molecular biology headed for what would soon grow in scope beyond that which few could then predict. Eiichi Soeda attended the meeting but did not openly discuss his country's plans. Soeda was in charge of a human genome sequencing project at the Riken Institute, Tokyo. Several well-known companies such as Fuji and Hitachi had started automating the sequencing process, which was predicted to reach the astonishing figure of 1 million bases a day within two years.

The Japanese Science and Technology Council had been supporting studies on a super DNA sequencing project since 1981, stressing development of robotic techniques. The plans envisioned DNA sequencing in a "sequencing factory" equipped with automated systems. Akyioshi Wada, a pioneer proponent of the Japanese human genome effort, intended that the sequencing should be coordinated at an international research center open to all researchers. He viewed the work as a chance for Japanese companies to use their well-known expertise in computers, electronics, and materials and sciences in the service of a biological project.

Soeda pointed out that while the sequencing was regarded as a very valuable end product, at least of equal importance was the improvement of biotechnology that would flow from the effort. The specter of Japanese superiority in the international biotechnology industry was perceived as a threat to the national self-interests of the United States. Visions arose of dedicated, efficient Japanese scientists utilizing high-tech instruments to win a race (not even officially begun) to sequence the entire human genome. As it turned out the Japanese soon became minor players in the growing international human genome effort led by the United States. However, this blend of scientific idealism and pure pragmatism flowing from the Cold Spring Harbor Symposium had generated a major controversy within the scientific community at all levels.

Meanwhile, DOE sought further guidance from its Health and Environmental Research Advisory Committee (HERAC). This committee is a group of scientists from universities, national laboratories, and private corporations that advises the Director of the Office of Energy Research on the science programs supported by the Office of Health and Environmental Research (OHER). In late 1986 HERAC put together a subcommittee on the human genome to make recommendations about what had come to be known as the DOE's "Human Genome Initiative." The subcommittee included members from the Howard Hughes Medical Institute, universities, biotechnology companies, and one from a national laboratory.

Their report of April 1987 urged DOE and the nation to commit to a major multidisciplinary effort. A new two-stage research effort should be created. The first (5–7 years) would emphasize generating physical chromosome maps, sequencing of selected DNA segments, and development of new methods of mapping and sequencing, that stressed automation and robotics. Also, computer methods, data base materials repositories, networks, and other resources to facilitate the process and best utilize its funding would have to be developed. The second phase would entail determining the complete sequence for each chromosome and making new techniques available for use in critical questions in medicine and biology. Because the science was of a "highly creative nature" they stressed that it should be widely distributed among universities, national laboratories, and private companies. The research should be a blend of small groups supported by investigator-initiated grants as well as large multidisciplinary centers.

The subcommittee offered as its primary rationale the potential utility of the initiative. The new techniques and the data that this research would produce would increase the efficiency of future improvements to human health and assist in the economic growth of industries dependent on biotechnology. The report concluded by warning against the danger of allowing this undertaking to interfere with the funding of worthwhile ongoing programs such as research on nonhuman organisms. Finally, the report recommended that the DOE have a leadership role in all this because of its history of successfully managing large multidisciplinary projects that involve the development of new technologies and in coordinating the mixture of national labs, universities, and private industries.

Once again a report had stressed the link between the mission of DOE to understand the health effects of radiation, which required detailed knowledge of the damage to the genome, and its initiation and support of numerous programs leading to technological developments. These seemed to make the DOE the logical agency for human genome mapping and sequencing. A budget of $20 million was proposed for the DOE Human Genome Initiative for fiscal year 1988 which would increase to $200 million by 1995. Congress eventually appropriated $10.7 million for that purpose for fiscal year 1988.

In September 1987 the Secretary of Energy issued a directive that established Human Genome Centers at the Los Alamos Laboratory and at the Lawrence Berkeley Laboratory to carry out research and technological development for flow-sorting of chromosomes, physical mapping, cloning, data management, and automated sequencing. The DOE program was well under way.

Ever since the proposal to map and sequence the human genome had gained momentum, discussions and dissent among biologists had centered about two themes—how such a project might be organized and how it would be funded. The DOE had not faltered in its intention to continue its genome initiative. The 1987 HERAC report had asserted that "DOE can and should organize and administer this initiative." DOE "should not delay implementation of its plan or defer to some other organization." The NIH, while eager to exert some influence on a project whose medical and scientific aspects were within their realm of interest and expertise, was nevertheless nervous about the scale and the potential to divert funds from other areas of research.

But what agency should take the lead? Should the focus be on complex genomes in general or exclusively on the human genome? Should the research be carried out in large research centers rather than the traditional, individual or small group approach? Congress was no doubt interested, particularly since they saw the results of this work as a way to give the United States a competitive edge in biotechnology and medicine. At the same time Congress was uneasy about appropriating substantial sums of money in a massive uncoordinated and possibly redundant method. A "Subcommittee on the Human Genome" was established by the Biotechnology Science Coordinating Committee (BSCC), a group which monitored biotechnology for President Reagan's domestic policy council.

The *Wall Street Journal* had left no doubt about its support for the advance of American biotechnology. In a June 1987 editorial, commenting on animal rights activists and environmentalists attacking fields where scientists were testing genetically engineered bacteria, they stated, "The issues raise the question of whether the United States will continue to be a world leader in scientific progress or whether groups of neo-Luddites will be able to impede that process under false theories of environmental concern and the 'rights' of nature. If this group succeeds in raising significant political barriers to United States science, the scientists will take their research and its benefits overseas . . . not knowing what science is doing makes it more likely that the no [sic]-nothings will retard the delivery of science's benefits to man."

As these discussions continued, by late 1987 it was unclear what exact shape DOE's project would take. Charles DeLisi, who had guided the effort at DOE, left to take on the chair of the Biomathematics Department at Mount Sinai School of Medicine, New York. And NIH, while encouraging research in new mapping and sequencing strategies and in the development of new data management systems had not yet committed themselves to an all-out effort.

Even before the HERAC subcommittee met to formalize a human genome initiative, within DOE a group of scientists had gathered in Woods Hole, Massachusetts at the world-renowned Marine Biology Laboratory. They began work on formulating a proposal for a study by the National Research Council (NRC). The NRC had been established in 1916 to provide advice to the federal government on science issues. At that time the emphasis was on the relevance of science in preparation for World War I. Since then its role had expanded to many other issues relating to science and technology.

The 15 member NRC committee had represented a wide spectrum of groups and included some that had voiced strong opposition to a large-scale expensive analysis of the human genome. The chairperson, Bruce Albert, had published articles in which he expressed doubts about the effectiveness of large research centers for large biological projects.

Despite the presence of skeptics, according to James Watson "soon after the NRC began its deliberations, it became apparent that within the meeting room the project itself was not really controversial—who could be against attaining the much higher resolution molecular genetic and physical maps of human DNA that would be needed to begin?" Among the committee members were scientists who had personal experience with mapping and sequencing DNA and appreciated the need first to emphasize the development of chromosome maps as invaluable tools for finding human disease genes.

In February 1988 the NRC committee released its report which unanimously urged a major commitment to a human genome project. They recommended that the federal funding should rise quickly to $200 million a year and that the project should be completed in approximately 15 years. A major concern had arisen during the discussions which would prove to be ultimately influential in shaping the future of human genome studies. The scientists' experience told them that an exclusive focus on the human DNA sequence might generate a great deal of information that would be all but uninterpretable without a comparable understanding of the genomes of less complex organisms such as yeast, the fruit fly, or the mouse. Experiments impossible with humans could be carried out with these organisms, and correlating sequences of their DNA with specific functions would make it much easier to infer the functions of similar genes in the humans. They recommended that sequencing such model genomes should be in parallel with or even ahead of that of the human genome.

Who would be in charge? The committee suggested that only one federal agency be in charge of organizing and coordinating the nation's effort in genome studies. They did not identify a particular agency but, according to Victor McCusick, "privately, however, many believed the lead agency should be the NIH because of its record in biomedical research both intramural and extramural."

Certainly the early enthusiasm for full-scale sequencing of the human genome first raised in public discussions at Cold Spring Harbor in the early summer of 1986 had evolved into a generally accepted, more modest initial goal of chromosomal mapping. A complete sequence of the genome's more than 3 billion bases had now become, in the committees words, " a subsidiary goal." Despite this well-documented shift in emphasis, the accusation that scientists were intent on seeking the sequence despite not knowing how to interpret it continues to dog their footsteps in press conferences and in public and private discussions.

A distinguished committee member was noticeably absent from the second meeting of the NRC committee. Harvard biologist Walter Gilbert, departing from what was turning into a power struggle between two major government agencies, NIH and DOE, had withdrawn from the committee to continue his plans to establish a private company, Genome Corporation. His company would, he stated boldly, "create a catalog of all human genes." The data would be put into a data base "where it would be made available to everyone for a price." He had been raising funds for this venture and though short of the $10 million in venture capital that he needed, he expected to be in business in mid-1987 with a company employing 200 people who would complete the sequence in about ten years.

Gilbert, a self-styled technological optimist, had with considerable chutzpah declared that he could copyright DNA sequences. His reasoning was: "someone worked it out and wrote it down—so the order of letters is copyrightable like a string of letters in a book."

True, molecular biologists were not strangers to the concepts of copyrights. Many already had corporate ties of some kind. And yet there were major objections to the prospect of someone "owning" the human genome. Frank Ruddle of Yale University, who had conducted gene mapping workshops in New Haven, Connecticut since 1973 felt that "being able to copyright the sequence would make me very uncomfortable." More directly, C. Thomas Caskey of Baylor University stated that "this information is so important that it cannot be proprietary. This is the first time we'll ever get this information on man—can we make a special case?"

Parallel with the work of the NRC panel, the Office of Technology Assessment (OTA) of the United States Congress was asked by the House Committee on Engineering and Commerce to prepare recommendations on genome studies. OTA's basic function is to help legislators to anticipate and plan for the results of technological changes and to examine the ways in which technology affects peoples' lives. This involves explaining the physical, biological, economic, social, and political impacts that can flow from applying scientific knowledge.

The OTA report, therefore, was couched in terms of options open to Congress. There was, however, no mistaking the message of the report. Some form of HGP was bound to continue and Congress should move it in the right direction, notably one that would secure United States leadership in what they recommended should be an international collaborative effort.

The report pointed out that NIH, DOE, NSF, and HHMI were already deeply involved in certain aspects of human genome research at various levels. It recommended against using the term "Human Genome Project," arguing that the term misrepresented the intent to develop methods applicable to all DNA. (This suggestion was ultimately to no avail as the term has persisted. It is used almost interchangeably with the "Human Genome Initiative," which technically refers to the DOE genome program.)

They stated that since "the agency most affected by genome projects will be the NIH," Congress might want to choose NIH as the lead agency. The other options raised were an interagency task force, a national consortium or (the least favored) simply congressional oversight. Their report pointed to the fact that NIH funds over ten times more genetic research than any other government or nongovernment organization. They stressed that should NIH be designated as the lead agency, it would have to recognize and coordinate with other genome activities at DOE, NSF, and other organizations.

The OTA report estimated the cost for mapping and sequencing for the first five-year period would start at $47 million in fiscal year 1989 and increase to $228 million by fiscal year 1993. The projection for fiscal year 1989 turned out to be approximately the amount that was appropriated for NIH and DOE, $27.6 and $17.5 million, respectively. The report admitted the long list of social and ethical implications that would need to be considered as part of policy analysis. These included issues ranging from the appropriate allocation of resources to much more complex questions concerning personal freedom, privacy, right of access to genetic information, and the possibility of applying genetic data to alter human disease, human talents, and human behavior. They noted that "the complexity and urgency of these issues will increase in proportion to advances in mapping and sequencing."

These issues were by no means to be resolved by the report, but many were relieved to see them at least described in part and alluded to as an official concern. Critics of the lack of progress in resolving such issues had already led biotechnology critic Jeremy Rifkin to create a coalition calling for more government attention on the ramifications of genome projects. Rifkin, long an outspoken activist against biotechnology, would later file suit to block gene transfer in humans. He was backed by a diverse assemblage of supporters including ethicists, labor leaders, insurance watchdog groups, consumer health advocates, and civil rights activists working for the establishment of a human genome policy board to advise Congress on the implications of such research.

Although in 1987 there was no formal request from NIH for genome studies in terms of a specific human genome project, during the spring of the 1987 House Appropriations hearings the then-director of NIH, James Wyngaarden, ventured the opinion that $50 million would be needed for a productive program. Later in May, James Watson and David Baltimore approached members of the House and Senate Appropriations Committee on behalf of the Delegation for Basic Biomedical Research. They emphasized the need for a several hundred million dollar increase in funding for AIDS research. They added that perhaps $30 million would allow NIH to begin a serious concerted genome program. Eventually Congress appropriated $17.2 million for that purpose for the fiscal year 1988.

As the results of the NRC report were made public, several thousand scientists gathered in Boston, Massachusetts for the annual meeting of the American Association for the Advancement of Science. Committee members who had drafted the NCR report were there to discuss its implications. They were adamant that the money to support a major genome program must not be at the expense of other biological research. David Botsein argued that "it will not work . . . if we take the resources away from something else." Arguing that he and many of his colleagues could not foresee garnering many benefits from the project he suggested that "the money would be better spent on AIDS research." James Watson countered that "we want thirty times more for AIDS than the genome."

Victor McCusick, Professor of Medical Genetics at Johns Hopkins University, Baltimore, maintained that funding would not falter because there would be spin-offs all along the way. "We don't have to wait for the whole map," he said, "we already have plenty of benefits." McCusick predicted that the project would eventually receive funding from international sources as well and spoke of plans to form an international genome organization to integrate research in the U.S., Europe, and Japan.

The appropriation of $17.2 million marked the formal involvement of NIH in the HGP. James Wyngaarden convened an 18-member "Ad Hoc Advisory Committee on Complex Genomes" to determine priorities for the NIH Genome Program. The board supported his proposal to establish an Office of Human Genome Research. The office was charged with overseeing the planning and operation of NIH-supported genome research and to coordinate NIH genome activities with other U.S. and international agencies. The new associate director began his duties in October of 1988. He was James Watson.

Many thought it fitting that the man who had literally helped to usher in the age of DNA research should oversee its logical conclusion. While critics suggested that the proposed 15-year goal for attaining the complete human DNA sequence more then coincidentally coincided with Watson's expectations for his professional life span, they could not deny that he had been an effective spokesperson for the project. Before his appointment he had argued that "a visible active scientist had to be in charge to reassure Congress, the general public and the scientific community that scientific reasoning, not the pork barrel, would be the dominant theme in allocating the soon to be larger genome monies."

Watson's effectiveness has perhaps been due as much to his heroic stature in the eyes of many as his scientific expertise. He has achieved the status of a cult figure. His name is known to anyone with even a cursory knowledge of science and while he can be gruff and outspoken, his colleagues have no choice but to respect his intellectual judgment. Watson, in agreeing to take on the task while continuing as Director of the Cold Spring Harbor Laboratory, "realized that only once would I have the opportunity to let my scientific life encompass the path from the double helix to the 3 billion steps of the human genome."

As the details of the evolving plans for the HGP spread out into the scientific journals and popular press the range of opposition broadened. An editorial titled "Genes Rampant" in *The Economist* continued to question the logic of seeking the entire human genome sequence. It warned of seeing "biology wholly in terms of genes" which would "be like studying Shakespeare word for word without feeling for the language . . . picking out the minutiae of a text is only one way of looking at literature; genetics is just one way of looking at life . . . people are not just bags of genes." Despite the fact that the complete human genome sequence had long since been relegated to the back burner as a primary goal, except by a few, and not a scientist worth his or her salt would ever suggest that people, him- or herself included, are just "bags of genes," the objections to "senseless sequencing" and reductionism would continue to be repeated.

Some respected scientists were equally concerned about large-scale sequencing. Robert Weinberg, whose own research depended on analyzing human genes for retinoblastoma, commented "I fear . . . that the important discussions have already been made and that the great sequencing juggernaut will soon begin its inexorable forward motion, flooding our desks with oceans of data whose scope defies conception and our ability to interpret meaningfully."

As genome research proceeded in parallel at DOE and NIH, Congress was faced with decisions of what its own role would be in the oversight and regulation of what promised to be a project of major proportions. Scientific, medical, and technological breakthroughs were already appearing and the public debate over the social, ethical, and legal ramifications was escalating.

Scientists, while more than happy to receive federal funding and thereby operate under federal guidelines, have traditionally preferred to trust their own expertise to guide the direction and details of their research. DOE and NIH had consistently stated that informal cooperation and coordination were all that was necessary to run the HGP. Congress, however, concerned about accountability and redundancy, appeared to be heading toward establishing formal interagency structures.

Apparently to head off a burdensome bureaucracy, NIH and DOE drafted a "Memorandum of Understanding" for interagency coordination. It was quickly signed by NIH's James B. Wyngaarden and Robert O. Hunter, Director of DOE's Office of Energy Research. The agreement called for a joint DOE/NIH "Subcommittee on the Human Genome" and for separate Joint Working Groups on mapping, informatics, and ethical, legal, and social issues. It also stressed coordination of efforts with other federal agencies and private organizations involved in related research. The subcommittee is made up of members of the NIH Program Advisory Committee on the Human Genome (PACHG), established by order of Congress in December 1988, and the DOE Health and Environmental Advisory Committee (HERAC). The 12-member subcommittee meets quarterly to provide overall scientific coordination. Its membership, chaired by Norton Zinder of the Rockefeller Institute, is drawn from universities, medical schools, and industries. Finally, the scientists of DOE and NIH had joined ranks. The two agencies with different skills and outlooks on the project were to complement each other well but the rivalry would remain.

The cover of the March 20, 1989 edition of *Time* featured an array of newborns surrounding the caption "Solving the Mysteries of Heredity: the drive to map human genes could revolutionize medicine but also raises troubling ethical questions." The cover story quotes Norton Zinder speaking to the Program Advisory Committee on the Human Genome (a "hushed audience"): "Today we begin." The article goes on to say "with these words spoken in January 1989, Zinder formally launched a monumental effort that could rival in scope both the Manhattan Project which created the A-bomb and the Apollo moon landing program—and may exceed them in importance."

Well, the analogies were by then quite familiar; but was this the official beginning of the HGP? According to Charles Cantor, spokesperson for the DOE, "there is no consensus as to when the HGP began." A convenient date for a "official" beginning is October 1, 1990, when the joint DOE/NIH five-year plan went into operation.

Certainly the January 1989 meeting achieved a consensus as to the immediate direction of the NIH approach. While the ultimate goal was still to map and sequence the human genome, they agreed that the work should begin with emphasis on other complex genomes such as the bacterium *E. coli*, yeast, roundworms, and the fruit fly *Drosophila*. This comparative genetic approach had finally reassured those who saw the generation of such a sequence unrelated to other information as a waste of time and money.

The committee also concluded that a principal aim would be to support research that promised to bring a three- to fivefold improvement in either knowledge or technology. This requirement would eventually change as the magnitude of the task became more apparent. By the end of 1990 at least a tenfold improvement in sequencing technology had become the goal, according to Charles Cantor. No one knew whether that would come from existing technology or the creation of new methods—if at all.

Undoubtedly the meeting marked the beginning of a new era in human genome studies. Research accelerated as the NIH human genome budget rose from $28.2 million in fiscal year 1989 to $59.5 million in fiscal year 1990 and $88 million in fiscal year 1991. In that same period the DOE human genome funding advanced from $18.5 million to $27.9 million to $46 million. As the HGP became a high-profile item in newspapers, periodicals, public radio, and television, critics from inside and outside the scientific community became more vocal.

A detailed history of this era would require a separate volume, but let's look at some of the principal events as they reflect on the progress and problems of those promising and often contentious times.

In late 1989 Charles Cantor, a prominent geneticist, was hired away from Columbia University to Lawrence Berkeley Laboratory to assume the directorship of the DOE Human Genome Center. He brought with him impressive scientific credentials as a member of the National Academy of Sciences, Associate Editor of the *Journal of Molecular Biology*, and author of a popular biophysical chemistry text. At Berkeley, Cantor and his co-workers continued with their mapping of chromosome 21.

In late April 1989, speaking in Washington, D.C., at a meeting jointly organized by the Alliance on Aging and the American Medical Association, James Watson suggested a plan to distribute responsibility for diverse chromosomes around the world. He suggested that in order to "just get the job done in the fastest time and at the lowest cost" that other countries be responsible not for doing all the research but "just for the coordination on the activities on a particular chromosome." Most disagreed. For instance, Sydney Brenner, U.K. Medical Research Council's Molecular Genetics Unit, warned that this would "balkanize" the human genome project.

The opposition to the plan was an opportunity to exacerbate the still simmering competition between DOE and NIH. Charles DeLisi, who had directed DOE's genome program, was now at Mount Sinai Medical Center. He commented that it is not a "science project, it's an engineering project" (and by implication more fitting for DOE). Senator Pete Domenici, R-New Mexico, a leading proponent for a larger role for DOE (Los Alamos is located in his state), told DOE Energy Research Director Robert Hunter at a May 1989 Senate Appropriations Subcommittee hearing: "You shouldn't settle for anything less than leadership in this field."

At this point in 1989 exactly where industry fit into the human genome effort remained uncertain. Several companies such as Applied Biosystems, Inc. (ABI, Redwood City, California) were specializing in genome-related technologies with the hope that their technological breakthroughs would become part of the mainstream of the government effort. Others concentrated on supplying instruments and reagents while still others looked forward to developing diagnostic and therapeutic approaches to the genetic diseases that were sure to be highlighted. Established companies such as Dupont (Wilmington, Delaware) took a long-term approach, according to Mark Pearson, a member of the NIH Advisory Committee and director of the company's molecular biology research. The company was "interested in the diagnosis of genetic and infectious disease . . . eventually drugs and protein products will come 20 or 30 years from now."

Some companies such as Collaborative Research (Bedford, Massachusetts) were already in the gene mapping business. Orrie Friedman, the company's chairperson and CEO, stated that developing a more refined map under federal auspices "will help us find disease genes, understand processes better, provide services to drug companies and even design drugs."

Testifying before the Congressional Subcommittee on International Scientific Cooperation on October 19, 1989, James Watson reasoned that "given the fact that every major country should be involved (in the HGP) it seems to me to make sense to try and reduce the final cost to the American public by having some form of sharing and so I have been an enthusiastic supporter of the formation of HUGO."

He was referring to the newly organized Human Genome Organization (HUGO) founded to further collaboration and cooperation in the worldwide genome effort. The founders, who included prominent scientists we have already mentioned in other contexts—Walter Bodmer, Frank Ruddle, Rento Dulbecco, Walter Gilbert and, yes, James Watson—had essentially appointed themselves as overseers of such diverse activities as the international linkage of data bases, advising governments on support for genome research, and monitoring of commercial and ethical issues. Dr. Victor McCusick was elected as the group's first president, quickly leading to a popular transformation of the organization's title as "Victor's HUGO." Despite being without official portfolio, by 1990 HUGO had grown to an elected membership of 350 prominent scientists from 23 nations.

Meanwhile, the *Wall Street Journal* again entered the fray in an editorial, complaining that "ethicists are worrying that such (genome) knowledge will exacerbate prejudices against individuals with 'non-normal' genes such as the handicapped or some unborn infants." The writer assured the readership that "surely an intelligent society should be able to cope with these issues while it pursued useful knowledge." That remained to be seen.

The editorial pointed up an issue that was of more concern, in their opinion. They agreed with David Baltimore of M.I.T. who had said that "megaprojects are inviting projects for the political control of science." Leaving no doubt as to where the *Wall Street Journal*, the so-called "bible of American business," stood, the editorial concluded that "the human genome initiative will be a strong test of the United States ability to shape and implement science policy. It will invite attack from those who are fearful or hostile toward the future. It should also attract the active support of those willing to defend the future."

Ethical issues related to genetic diseases continued to generate discussion and debate. In July 1989 a symposium entitled "Human Genetic Information: Science, Law and Ethics" met in Bern, Switzerland. Specialists in law, ethics, and theology reviewed diverse questions, for example, the results of identifying through genome analysis people who were likely to develop a serious disease long before the symptoms appear. Diana Brahams, a specialist in law related to medicine, warned that the information could be "of considerable interest to prospective employers, insurers, marriage partners, or family members and would be of serious concern to the individual." Speaking of the possibility of the introduction of genes for "desirable" characteristics such as athletic ability into human fertilized eggs, Bernard Davis of Harvard Medical School said "even if we find such use trivial, a world that accepts cosmetic surgery, the injection of silicone to enlarge breasts . . . may find it difficult to limit nonmedical uses." The feasibility of this manipulation for such trivial purposes was discounted by most scientists at the meeting.

Writing in the *Hastings Center Report*, George J. Annas, widely respected professor of health law at Boston University School of Medicine, took direct aim at the serious legal and ethical questions surrounding the HGP. He pointed out that mapping and sequencing the human genome could lead to genetic testing for not only diseases but even tendencies toward disease with unforeseeable consequences. He raised again the issue of information control and privacy, warning that employers, insurance companies, and the government, among others, would want to have access to the information contained in our genome. "Scientists might want such information restricted but they have little influence over its use . . . we are utterly unprepared for issues of mandatory screening, confidentiality, secrecy and discrimination. . . . Ethics is generally taken seriously by physicians and by scientists only when it either furthers their agenda or does not interfere with it."

One month later, in October 1989, Human Genome I convened in San Diego, California. It was billed as the first international gathering on the genome project. In its sweep and scope the HGP had become hard to describe even for scientists close to it. The *Wall Street Journal* quoted Daniel Koshland, editor of *Science* and co-chairperson of the conference: "Nothing Groucho Marx ever did is as zany as the HGP . . . it's a unique social experiment—controlled chaos." He warned that the possibility of compiling genetic information on individuals would require confidentiality and caution aided by legislation to prevent abuses.

In a *Science* editorial, planned to coincide with Human Genome I, Koshland, while admitting "there were immoralities of commission to avoid" admitted "there is also the immorality of omission—the failure to apply a great new technology to aid the poor, the infirm, and the underprivileged." Examples of just how these unfortunates were to be helped were not included.

In the same month NIH upgraded the Office of Human Genome Research to the National Center for Human Genome Research (NCHGR). James Watson continued as the director. By early the next year the center had a staff of 30 including Eric T. Juengst, who was hired by the NCHGR to run its program on ethical, legal, and social implications of human genome research. Juengst had previously served as bioethics consultant to the NRC during the preparation of its report and later the OTA panel examining genetic testing in the workplace. He oversees administration of grants to researchers in ethics and social policy, and coordinates NCHGR research with recommendations from the NIH and DOE working group on Ethical, Legal, and Social Issues (ELSI) chaired by Nancy

Wexler of Columbia University. In addition, he acts as a liaison between NCHGR and international groups involved in the same issues.

James Watson, soon after he became Director of the Office of Human Genome Research at NIH, had emphasized that at least 3% of the earmarked genome funds should be expended in support of ethics and social implications, stating that "if we fail to act now we might witness unwanted and unnecessary abuses that eventually will create a strong popular backlash against the human genetic community." However, one of Watson's closest associates remarked that "there is a vigorous debate within the genome scientist community about the wisdom of supporting ethical, legal, and social analysis and if you took a vote my guess is that it would be 60–40 or more against Watson."

The 89-page joint DOE/NIH report "Understanding Our Genetic Inheritance: The U.S. Human Genome Project: The First Five Years (FY 1991–1995)" was published in April 1990. It precisely stated the scientific goals for the first five years, as we have discussed in our treatment of mapping and sequencing. In addition, it clearly summarized the goals for informatics and ethics, complementary inputs of both agencies, described collaboration between U.S. and international groups, and offered budget projections.

No sooner was the plan in the hands of the scientific community than a grass roots effort was under way to stop the HGP. Martin Rechsteiner, a biochemist at the University of Utah School of Medicine, sent a letter to 500 scientists calling the project "mediocre science, terrible science policy." His major concern was that the HGP would surely divert funds from the rest of biology. Michael Syvanen, a bacterial geneticist at the University of California–Davis, publicized a letter, co-signed by five colleagues, which predicted the diversion of funds from more "diverse, inspired and problem-related research."

By June, Francis Collins, the co-discoverer of the cystic fibrosis gene and an active participant in the genome project, warned that "we have PR problem of major proportions." Watson and other leading scientists flocked to Capitol Hill to lobby for the proposed HGP NIH budget of $108 million. Bernard Davis of Harvard Medical School, and almost all the members of Harvard's Department of Microbiology and

Molecular Genetics, had joined the dissenters. Norton Zinder, chairperson of the NIH Program Advisory Committee on the Human Genome, lamented "why do they so completely misunderstand what we are about?"

Two months before Human Genome II convened in San Diego in late October 1990, Charles Cantor was removed as the head of the DOE Human Genome Center at Lawrence Berkeley Laboratory. The official explanation offered was that Cantor was being moved to a new position as principal scientist for the entire DOE genome effort. Those close to the scene alleged that Cantor's role as globe-trotting spokesperson had left little time for the day-to-day management of the lab. Relatively little had been accomplished on the chromosome 21 map, and the pressure to produce had led officials to initiate the search for a top-ranked scientist. Cantor, indeed an articulate and effective representative for DOE, allegedly had fallen victim to a timetable which was inexorably committed to progress.

The dust had barely settled when the genome conference opened, where to the surprise of many of the over 600 participants, two of the prominent critics of the HGP appeared on the speaker's program for the opening session. Bernard Davis from Harvard and Don Brown of the Carnegie Institution had been invited to make their case. Despite the three days of glowing reports of the scientific progress that had been made since Human Genome I, the calculated move to invite the enemy into the camp may have served to further publicize their growing disagreements.

Though roundly scolded by Walter Gilbert as essentially being out of the mainstream of molecular biology, unaware of a "paradigm shift" that had taken place, Davis and Brown gamely defended their positions. Although they made few converts, if any, in that congregation of scientists with a stake in the HGP, their objections and those of others not invited to speak with different agendas would have to be faced in the laboratories, clinics, and public forums of the future.

10

BIG SCIENCE, BAD SCIENCE?

Walter Bodmer, Director of Research at the Imperial Cancer Research Fund in London, is fond of describing the HGP as an extraordinary opportunity to gain an understanding of the genetic basis of disease. These new insights will lead to the possibility of developing methods of diagnosis and treatment. He speaks also of the way in which it will enable us to understand our origins and evolution. James Watson regards the HGP as a "public good" whose "principal goal is to assist biomedical researchers in their assault on disease . . . to better understand the afflictions that exact an enormous toll of human suffering on every culture and every geographic region."

Who could object to an undertaking defined by spokespersons of such renown? Who could find fault with a project whose aims are arguably in the best interests of humanity? The answer is, as indicated in the previous chapter, a wide spectrum of people with a correspondingly wide variety of agendas. The questions that they have raised have developed out of concerns which range from philosophical disagreement over the way scientific research ought to be carried out to serious ethical and societal issues such as genetic testing of populations, confidentiality, and gene therapy.

Not all of these issues are of equal significance, nor are the dilemmas that they raise equally tractable. Many of them, such as those that revolve around prenatal and postnatal diagnosis of genetic disease or even predisposition to such disease, genetic counseling, or the confidential nature of one's own genetic information, are not unique to the HGP. However, they have undoubtedly been brought into sharper focus because

235

of it. There are those who argue that the HGP does not raise any unique issues. They prefer to regard the issues in the words of Daniel Koshland as "old problems revisited . . . the information in the genome adds accuracy and scope to many of these applications but no new or threatening principles." Others would respond that it is this very "accuracy and scope" of the new genetic information that will undoubtedly flow from the HGP that will create problems different not just in degree but in kind. A host of ethical and legal issues are coming into focus. Koshland, in the same *Science* editorial, did admit that "if the higher visibility of the genome project causes a qualitative change then of course new procedures may be needed."

It is not our intention to try offer easy solutions to these complex controversies. We can best contribute to their ultimate resolution by first defining them as they relate specifically to the HGP and then clarifying them by reducing them where possible to the principles upon which they operate.

If one listens to the comments from the scientific community and reads the scientific literature, one is struck by the fact that criticisms of the HGP generally fall into two categories, neither of which has to do with strictly ethical issues. We are not aware of any concerted efforts within the scientific community to stop or interfere with human genome studies because of ethical concerns. That is not to suggest that scientists are not aware of the societal dilemmas which the HGP will generate. As we will describe in Chapter 11 in more detail, the DOE and the NIH have an active and expert Joint Working Group on Ethical, Legal, and Social Issues that studies the implications of mapping and sequencing the human genome. James Watson has insisted that these issues get a full public hearing. Three percent of the NIH budget, which over 15 years could be up to $90 million, is to be devoted to their study and resolution. Still, "ethics by committee" has its own peculiar problems, as we shall see.

Scientists generally center their criticisms of the HGP on two related themes. First, how can good scientific research best be accomplished? Second, how should this research be funded? No one argues with the ends, but the battles are fierce over the means.

What might seem like an esoteric subject fit for armchair philosophers of science actually has become a very contentious issue—the question of how best to conduct scientific research to maximize its potential for success, minimize the associated bureaucracy, and avoid unnecessary expense. In fact, this is the question that is really behind what is called the "big science" issue. "Big science" refers to a massive, long-term, and expensive scientific research program with strictly defined goals. If bigger science were always better science, then it follows that bigger science should be supported. But is the HGP big, and if so is it better?

"BIG SCIENCE"

The Manhattan Project, the Apollo Project, the Superconducting Supercollider (SSC), and the NASA Space Station Project have, as emblems of big science all been applied as parallels to the HGP. Media accounts of the HGP seem to favor these references *ad nauseam*. Such comparisons are repeated with equal frequency by both proponents and opponents for very different reasons. Some of the initiators and leaders of the HGP apparently feel that linking it to these massive efforts, heavily funded by the U.S. government and supported by the American taxpayers as triumphs of American know-how and international leadership, will endow it with continued acceptance and support, particularly with Congress.

Its detractors use the analogies to insinuate, among other things, that the HGP is inordinately expensive. They fear that it will tend to develop a life of its own which will eat up funds for other worthwhile research in the biological sciences. Calling it "super science, super expensive" a *New York Times* editorial referred to the HGP as "rococo" research which had one thing in common with the space station and the SSC: a "near total disregard of how such ventures might further American competitiveness."

Even more caustic was the interpretation of Robert Wright expressed in *The New Republic*: "by the mid 1980s the Department of Energy's ostensible mission of making nuclear weapons and making energy policy was sinking on the nation's agenda. Someone there had the resourcefulness to ask Congress for lots of money to do the Human Genome Project."

Some escape the contradictions inherent in the analogies by denying the analogies' validity. Renato Dulbecco, who had inspired James Watson's early interest in the HGP, contends that the "big science" label for the HGP is inappropriate. On the other hand, Charles Cantor accepts the "big science" label but argues that unlike other types of "big science" "this project is guaranteed to succeed . . . it is not basic research in any sense . . . it is engineering to provide a tool that will be used by people in basic research." Leroy Hood, who later was expected to succeed Charles Cantor in 1991 as the Director of the DOE Human Genome Center, argues that "Rather than big science, it is interdisciplinary science."

During his address at Human Genome II James Watson dismissed the criticisms against the HGP as "big science" by stating that "well, the human genome is big . . . I never thought that big was necessarily bad." Arguing that "most people would rather go to a big hospital than a small one" he went on to reassure the listeners that "we are not planning on building a secret DNA city somewhere." Having managed to beg the question by these remarks he then went straight to the heart of the matter. "We want it to be big enough so that the cost can be brought down to a reasonable level . . . (and) we want to get it done in a reasonable period of time . . . we shouldn't be fighting among ourselves."

On the other hand, Daniel Koshland, speaking before Watson, preferred to assert that the HGP "is small science compared to those others . . . it is big science to biologists who are mom and pop entrepreneurs." He pointed out that "If they [the SSC and the Space Station] were stopped halfway we would have essentially no information . . . the HGP if stopped in the middle—I don't recommend this—we would still have a great deal of information . . ."

In contrast, Walter Bodmer describes the HGP as "the most exciting science . . . more so than all these space shots and Hubble telescopes that have slight distortions in them so you can't see clearly . . . that distortion would have paid for the HGP . . . the Supercollider could pay for a few HGPs." Remember, Sir Walter Bodmer answers to Parliament and not to the U.S. Congress. When competing for funds on Capitol Hill, it is best not to criticize other programs with hat in hand for one's own.

Simply in terms of money the "big science" analogy actually puts the HGP in a good light. At its projected cost of $3 billion, the other "big science" projects dwarf it. The largest engineering project in the world, the Superconducting Supercollider, will be housed within a 54-mile-long circular tunnel carved out beneath the prairie of central Texas. It is designed to smash atomic particles together, simulating conditions at the birth of the universe—the so-called "Big Bang." Questions that have puzzled physicists for many years about the nature of matter and the evolution of the universe may be resolved—at a cost of $8 billion. On an even grander scale the Space Station, planned as a permanently occupied orbital laboratory, will cost $40 billion to construct and perhaps $80 billion to operate.

The analogies become less comfortable when one looks at the controversies generated by these megaprojects. For example, the plans for a supercollider were first broached in 1983. By 1987 the DOE had 43 site proposals for what promised to be an economic windfall for the state with a powerful enough lobby to capture it. Texas, with its adopted son George Bush on his way to the White House, won out. The SSC promises to bring thousands of jobs and billions of dollars to Texas, but economic impact studies also predict that the SSC debt service will create a $68.3 million annual deficit during the 20 years that it will operate.

After 20 years it will have to be abandoned because the tunnel will be dangerously radioactive. The local residents' fears of escape of radioactivity from the massive tunnel are not assuaged by assurances from the DOE. Recent disclosure of the years of radioactive contamination at the Rocky Flats nuclear weapons plant and Hanford and Savannah River nuclear reactors, all of which fall under the supervision of the DOE, have done little to allay their misgivings.

As far as the space station is concerned, 28 payloads of parts will have to be launched aboard the periodically troubled space shuttle. Astronauts will have to assemble the football-field-sized facility while floating high over the atmosphere tethered to their spacecraft. As one space station insider who asked to remain anonymous stated in a *Science* interview, "the work that's been done to date is crap" and "its not even good engineering." The station has gone through several major design changes and has apparently turned out to be a nightmare of logistics.

The *New York Times*, on another occasion, compared these two problematic projects, the SSC and the space station, with the "pharaohs of Egypt wasting their nations resources on shiny mortuary extravagances ignoring the steady decline of their civilization." Perhaps these are not the best analogies to perpetuate.

If that is not enough guilt by association, consider the analogies from yet another perspective. The Manhattan Project, the Apollo Project to land a man on the moon, the SSC, and the space station were all designed to varying degrees for military purposes.

The extraordinary scientific *tour de force* of the Manhattan Project, which unleashed the power of the atom, was accomplished by brilliant physicists and engineers. The fearsome demonstration of the theories about the properties of the atom was the epitome of twentieth-century physics. Yet it led to the deaths of hundreds of thousands in Hiroshima and Nagasaki. It has made possible the threat of the annihilation of civilization within minutes by accidental or intentional launching of nuclear warheads now poised in missile silos under the peaceful earth.

The Apollo Project, as George Annas so succinctly put it in the *Hastings Center Report*, "was about neither the inevitability of scientific advance nor the control of nature. Instead it was about military advantage and commercialism disguised as science and hyped as a peace mission." The nations of the world have been in a race to take the high ground in a military, not a moral, sense. The high ground of space gives a tactical advantage to those encamped there.

Robert Barker, assistant to the Secretary of Defense in 1987, wrote to the White House Domestic Council "the SSC project will have many spin-offs for the Department of Defense . . . especially in technologies required by the Strategic Defense Initiative including particle beams, information processing, computer control, pulse power sources, and high energy accelerators."

Perhaps the most unfortunate association of the HGP is that which links it to the Manhattan Project. According to Robert Oppenheimer, testifying before Congress in 1945, "When you come right down to it the reason we did this job [the Manhattan Project] is because it was an organic necessity. You can't stop such a thing. If you are a scientist you believe that it is good to find out how the world works; that it is good to find what the realities are; that it is good to turn over to mankind at large the greatest possible power to control the world . . ."

Walter Bodmer, in defending the participation of the U.K. in the HGP, similarly said "the first answer I would give is that the HGP is exciting science in which we ought to be involved by that criterion alone."

In both cases brilliant scientists have been driven by a search for knowledge whose pragmatic effects transcend that knowledge. In the wartime research in which Oppenheimer played a leading role, control over certain of the forces locked within the atom was achieved. It was an intellectual, scientific, and engineering triumph. It quickly became a tool of political and national power.

Many are concerned that the power to control the genes of living organisms, which has just begun to be achieved, will continue to expand dramatically as the HGP uncovers the location and nature of human genes. They fear that the use of this knowledge will prove to be beyond the control both of the scientists who have made the discoveries and that of society itself.

For example, the deeper our understanding becomes of the human genome, the greater is the possibility of using that understanding to create weapons for biological warfare. This is not a subject which is widely discussed in relation to the HGP but we are sure that increased attention will be paid to it. Charles Piller and Keith R. Yamamoto, in their 1988 book *Gene Wars–Military Control over the New Genetic Technologies*, point out, while not referring specifically to the HGP, that discoveries about the genetics of the human immune system might allow the engineering of viruses that would target that system and leave the victim defenseless against infection. Genes that direct the synthesis of hormones that regulate our moods, perceptions, body temperature, or other essential processes might be used to manufacture massive quantities of these substances.

Will we know that this is being done? Only if our government chooses to tell us. Once again, we are faced with the distinction between the search for knowledge and the uses to which that knowledge is put.

One would think that the HGP, which is being promoted as an

avenue to a new world of genetic medicine, with promises of diagnosis and treatment of devastating diseases, should make it a policy to discourage comparisons with highly controversial examples of "big science."

Whether or not the HGP should qualify as "big science" will continue to be argued. Terminology aside, the underlying question remains: Is the science of the HGP, big or not, to be judged as good science? That is, is the HGP the most efficient, productive, and cost-effective way to analyze the human genome? We have combined here the arguments of a number of critics, all of whom are scientists. Not all would defend each of these positions. The arguments against the HGP being good science go as follows.

"GOOD SCIENCE?" NO!

The United States has had a proud history of accomplishment in the biological and medical sciences. We have gained extraordinary insights into the structure and function of living organisms from the subcellular level to the behavior, evolution, and ecology of populations. This progressively deeper understanding of the living world has resulted in, for example, an increased human life span and control over many infectious diseases which have plagued humans for centuries. The development of vaccines, antibiotics, and other pharmaceuticals has freed many humans from suffering which even in recent history had seemed inevitable.

In addition, our increasing knowledge of how organisms contribute to and interact with each other in their physical environment has enabled us to better realize ways in which to practice stewardship over increasingly threatened planetary ecosystems. For example, we can now more competently document the damage done to living systems by such phenomena as the destruction of the rain forests, the pollution of the oceans, or the indiscriminate use of pesticides and herbicides.

These advances have come out of an approach to experimental science that places its confidence in investigator-initiated research. This means that it has been left up to the individual scientist first to determine what he or she considers an important question to ask, and then to develop a proposal for monetary support for that research which is reviewed and judged by scientific peers. Often, but certainly not always, the research has led to unexpected findings in addition to answers to the original questions. These results, once reported in the literature, have been used by other investigators in fruitful ways never envisioned by their discoverers. After all, who would have guessed that yeast or roundworms had genes that were identical to those in humans? Who would have thought that restriction enzymes isolated from simple bacteria would make genetic engineering possible?

This seemingly random approach to scientific questions has in fact been the pride of American science. It is a so-called "bottom up" approach, where the ideas are left to the scientist as well as the means by which these ideas are to be carried out in the laboratory or in the field. In this traditional and highly successful system scientists investigate what they consider important, not what someone tells them is important. The opposite "top down" approach as exemplified by the HGP turns what has been a creative, productive system into a monolithic project which tells the scientists what is to be accomplished, when the results are due, and suggests ways in which it can be done.

Research which is top down or "targeted" tends to need a larger budget than the traditional or "nontargeted" approach. It also involves a complicated and thereby more expensive administrative bureaucracy which has to micromanage the project.

Another problem with targeted research is that it tends to attract mediocre people who otherwise might not have been funded. The training of graduate students, our future scientists, is perverted by emphasizing technique-oriented work—mapping, sequencing—in place of the milieu in which learning to ask questions and devising experiments to answer them is the most valuable lesson. The more creative scientists are thus left behind for the more proficient technician.

If those that have led the fight for separate HGP funds had instead hidden the project within the ordinary individual grant procedures of the NIH, it would have had less visibility and would not have come under attack. It also might have resulted in a broader approach to genetics. Perhaps they should have used their influence to create a diffuse program which would include DNA sequencing as just one way to get to the disease-carrying genes. For example, perhaps it would be better to first look for the proteins that these genes are producing and work backward from the biochemistry of the protein to the RNA that helped put it together and finally to the gene. We admit that much AIDS research has been targeted and effective—but AIDS is a national emergency.

Further, the HGP has already funded four multidisciplinary research centers and plans to increase that number to at least 20 over the next few years both at universities and at private companies. These are to be special centers, each with up to 25 scientists and technicians. That means that up to half of the money designated for genome research will go to these centers. This changes the whole social fabric of science. The people in these centers will be working on sharply focused objectives, for example, the sequence of yeast. Productive science has seldom been done that way. Centers are expensive to set up and maintain. Even if they are not performing up to expectations, which is itself difficult to determine, it is difficult to close them down.

Actually, once the outline of what needs to be done is clear, most of the work involved in creating a physical map and sequencing will not be creative or insightful science. It will be technicians' work, repetitive, mind numbing, and not attractive to bright Ph.D.s or graduate students.

Also, between 95 to 98% of human DNA consists of what is commonly called "junk DNA." This does not give information to the cell and probably has no function at all. The genes that are causing genetic disease are located on the remaining 2 to 5% of the genome. These can be located and sequenced without sequencing the entire genome. Thus a great deal of time and money is wasted by not concentrating efforts on this relatively small amount of useful DNA.

This disruptive departure from a research methodology which has proven to be effective actually is retarding the attainment of disease prevention and possible cure. It is a roadblock to progress in American science and technological development.

As you can see, many of the arguments against the HGP strike deeper than merely complaints against techniques. They question the very validity of its approach to science. Those who disagree with these

critics—again we are combining the rebuttals of a number of proponents—might answer the earlier detractors as follows.

"GOOD SCIENCE?" YES!

The HGP is good science. In fact, it's the scientists themselves that
want to do it this way. The traditional method of investigator-initiated
research is not the only way to do science. Besides, that traditional
approach has not furnished effective answers to major diseases such as
cancer, which the HGP is particularly suited to address. We need to target
the disease genes and we now know how to get to them—by mapping and
sequencing.

Can we give up this organized search, the top down targeted
approach, which we hope will lead to diagnosis and eventually treatment
and leave it up to chance that someone will decide to work on these
projects? Why take the chance of duplicating efforts when one can
prevent redundancy by supervising large numbers of people who are
working within the same program?

The HGP has attracted skilled, creative scientists as evidenced by
the progress made so far. The idea that graduate students are never
assigned projects but are always independent, creative scientists is
inaccurate. There is room for both targeted and nontargeted research.
Both can be productive and offer good training for prospective scientists.

Somehow "hiding" the genome program within the ordinary NIH
budget would not have raised sufficient funding for it nor would it have
had the visibility and coordination needed to attract good scientists and
their research without the well-defined major goals of the HGP. Remember, the HGP does include a broad approach to genetics. We are already
looking at the genomes of a number of organisms in detail such as
bacteria, yeast, worms, and mice.

To argue that we should look first for proteins and then trace back to
the genes that produce them is out of date. To be sure this is often
effective, but modern molecular techniques make a direct large-scale and
integrated assault on the genome by mapping and sequencing, a more

powerful tool for a more rapid, productive, and precise way of finding and analyzing greater number of genes.

Since the HGP has as its published short-term goals physical maps of human and other genomes, it is inaccurate to suggest that we are encouraging "senseless" sequencing. Research toward improvement of sequencing technology is being supported but unless there is a major breakthrough in the speed and cost of sequencing it will not be done on a large scale.

Research centers are necessary in order to get the job done quickly and efficiently. If the goal of the HGP were the usual NIH "cottage industry" approach, it would take 100 years to get the sequence of the human genome. The HGP does not take away opportunities for the traditional approach, it simply creates a new way to answer important questions. The centers will be reviewed three years after they are set up to monitor their efficiency.

True, much of the work of mapping and sequencing is repetitive. But with advances in automation already being developed more of this can be done by technicians who are used to monitoring machines. This will liberate senior investigators for more creative work. After all, its not just sequencing but rather deciding what to sequence that takes expertise.

As far as "junk DNA" is concerned, that is a misnomer. We do not know what importance these sequences hold. A better term would be Harvard's Bernard Davis's suggestion "terra incognita." It's bad science to assume that these areas of the genome have no value until we study them thoroughly.

As scientists we know that organisms are more than just DNA and the proteins for which it codes. But we also know that the life of the cell and hence that of the organism is dependent on the proper functioning of its genes. We have a world of understanding about those basic life functions in health and disease waiting to be explored. The most rapid, efficient, and cost-effective way to do this is through the HGP.

Despite the debate over what is certainly a fundamental dichotomy of opinion over the way science ought to be carried out, would this debate be so intense if enough money were available to fund adequately the research of all the participants in the debate? We have used the term "small science" and "cottage industry" approach; but to set up even a small state-of-the-art molecular biology laboratory requires at least $50,000 to $100,000. Most of this money comes from federal funding agencies.

FUNDING

In 1991, the first fiscal year of the DOE/NIH five-year plan, the NIH National Center for Human Genome Research received a line item appropriation of $88 million out of a total NIH appropriation of $7.98 billion. A year earlier human genome research at NIH was awarded $59.5 million as compared to $28.2 million in 1989. The total NIH budget for those years was $7.5 billion in fiscal year 1990 and $7.2 billion in fiscal year 1989.

Behind what seems like a hefty increase for both the HGP and funding for other research as well, there is the specter of Gramm–Rudman. The Gramm–Rudman Deficit Reduction Act of 1985 sets a target which the government must try to meet. Unless Congress comes within $10 billion of that figure, automatic across-the-board cuts go into effect. In 1989, for example, Congress failed to reach the $10 billion target which resulted in cuts of 1.7%, removing tens of millions of dollars from the NIH budget. In 1991, the target was $64 billion. There is developing, as a congressional Budget Office analyst said, "a definite squeeze in discretionary programs."

Meanwhile at NIH, only 4700 new grants were funded in 1990 compared to 6500 two years before. Judgments about the merits of grant applications are made by "study sections," each of which specializes in a particular area of science. Among the grants recommended for support by the study sections, the fraction actually funded had fallen from more than 40% to less than than 25%. Also, to spread the limited funds, NIH cut the budgets of all awarded grants by 10 to 20% from recommended levels.

In practical terms, according to Bernard Davis, "study sections thus face the depressing prospect of virtually tossing a coin to choose among scientists with a continuing record of distinguished achievement and promising beginners are even more at risk." This has the unfortunate result of interrupting the continuity of what is often good research while discouraging bright students from seeking careers in science.

Martin Rechsteiner, professor and co-chairperson of the Department of Biochemistry at the University of Utah School of Medicine, is more direct. Writing about the HGP in 1990, he declared that "in the worst funding year for decades we see a proposal to distribute previously unheard of amounts of money to a handful of scientists . . . a small group of established scientists will command very large amounts of money while numerous young scientists are currently unfunded." He pointed out that $200 million represents more than 1000 research grants—about seven grants for each major research university in the United States. He concluded that "we are wasting money on big ticket items while our science infrastructure is collapsing."

Michael Syvanen, a professor of microbiology and immunology at the University of California at Davis, is another outspoken critic. He, like Rechsteiner, has been engaged in a letter-writing campaign to stop the HGP. He asserts that "no one takes seriously anymore the original claim that the HGP will not drain funds from the rest of biological science." Further, he claims that "there is general agreement among responsible scientists that the very goals that the Human Genome Initiative claims—the curing of human disease—will be actually hurt because more medically relevant and effective research programs will be unfunded."

The *New York Times* reports that in "dozens of interviews with experts in and out of government the message was loud and clear." Small-scale research is being "squeezed," "in crisis," "dying." In the same edition Dr. Richard S. Nicholson, Executive Director of the American Association for the Advancement of Science, stated that "there is really a high level of discouragement and distress in the scientific community . . . if you go around and talk to this country's top scientists they're about to bag it."

What are the answers to these criticisms and concerns? The organizers of the HGP maintain that this program has quite simply received funding as a separate item and it has not taken financial support from other areas of research. They cite the increase in the NIH budget from year to year as indicating that Congress has not siphoned money from traditional programs to bolster the HGP.

James Watson, in his usual outspoken manner, stated in a National Public Radio interview that "there is panic in the scientific community so they want to blame someone. They can't blame the fact that lots of money is going to AIDS because then it looks like its against all sorts of minority groups so they take it out on us."

The difficulty with this defensive stance is a problem faced by the critics as well. Both sides, at least those who are willing to go beyond assertions, admit that neither side can actually offer incontrovertible evidence to prove its position. Bernard Davis, in his address at Human Genome II, admitted that there was no way to give a precise proof of this competition but "in a time of financial crisis the most important [factor] is the bottom line according to Congress." In a freewheeling press conference later that day, Daniel Koshland pointed out that no one could actually prove that the HGP was interfering with other funding. Don Brown of the Carnegie Institution in Washington, D.C., speaking of a serious crunch in investigator-initiated grants along with a rapid increase in HGP funding, argued that it "is almost self-evident that there is competition." In an earlier *New York Times* interview Davis had stressed "[I] just can't prove it; but, I think that it is widely felt that the two are in competition."

While neither side can prove its point beyond a doubt it is clear that there has developed a widespread sense that the HGP represents a feast among famine. As the Gramm–Rudman strictures continued to be applied and the demand by qualified scientists for funding continues to far exceed the supply, the work of the participants in meeting the announced goals of the HGP will come under increasing scrutiny by the scientific community as well as Congress.

One of the very unfortunate consequences of what has been described as a "feeding frenzy" for funds is that it has set scientist against scientist. Leon M. Lederman, director of the Fermi National Accelerator Laboratory, has suggested that what is needed instead is "a grand unification of scientists with the conviction that what is good for science is good for the nation." He appeals to scientists to "marshal forces, link arms, raise banners and insist that science may be the last hope of humanity." Lederman suggests that $2 billion per year could meet the needs of all nonmilitary, university-based science research.

We are not sure that the image of a phalanx of scientists who, as he adds, can lead us to "a human destiny, a golden age out there" would be effective in an era when much about science is either not understood or even feared, but he raises a point well worth considering. Looked at from the perspective of what the U.S. government is willing to spend on military research and development, the budgetary requests for medical research in general, let alone the HGP, can be regarded as almost begging for scraps from a plentiful table. After all, one Trident submarine costs $1.4 billion. The Stealth bomber program is estimated at $68 billion while the requested SDI funding for fiscal years 1988–1992 is $38 billion.

Nobel laureates argue vociferously over how to distribute sums which are minute fractions of the price of these weapons systems whose purpose is to destroy human life. Six months of U.S. outlays for nuclear warheads is greater than the total estimated $3 billion cost of the entire projected 15-year Human Genome Program, whose purpose is to understand life itself more deeply.

In testimony before Parliament on January 23, 1990, Walter Bodmer noted that "At this time, when there is a remarkable easing of tension between East and West politically, and when one can hope that there is less need to expend the extraordinary amount that we do on our defence systems so that more resources can become available for other areas of human endeavour, I would put the Human Genome Project at the top of my list of priorities." Perhaps American scientists will become more vocal on this question which, if resolved in favor of nonmilitary investment, might render questions of "big science" and "good science" obsolete.

INTERNATIONAL

The scope of the international effort of the HGP was clearly in evidence at the Human Genome II conference in October 1990. Of the 180 lectures and poster presentations at this symposium, 46 were authored by scientists from outside the United States. Of course, genetic studies have never been the exclusive province of one country. A wide international network of collaborators has been collaborating in the study of the genetics of cystic fibrosis, Huntington's disease, Alzheimer's disease, Duchenne muscular dystrophy, and many other diseases.

In addition to the United States, the U.K., the U.S.S.R., Italy, and Japan have organized human genome programs. Plans are underway for programs in France, Canada, the People's Republic of China, and Australia. The European Community has started a 35-laboratory, six-year, $20 million effort to sequence small genomes, beginning with that of yeast. Italy supports a $1.3 million per year effort while the Medical Research Council in the U.K. initiated a three-year, $22 million genome program in 1989 which is predicted to increase to $40 million. The U.S.S.R. was investing $36 million by 1990. Japan has initiated several genome-related research undertakings which had reached a total of approximately $8 million by 1990. Britain's efforts, which are concentrating on mapping the human genome with emphasis on disease genes, is particularly intensive and marked by a long-term commitment.

John Galloway, head of public relations at the Cancer Research Campaign in London, explained in *New Scientist* that the importance of Britain's participation was in the fact that "whoever gets the human genome data first will decide what will happen to them [the data] and will be in an unassailable position to dictate terms over its commercial, including its medical exploitation. . . . Britain has to buy itself a seat at the international bargaining table and we will probably have less than five years to establish our credentials . . . bidding will not wait for the project to be completed, it will start as soon as there is anything worth selling."

Somehow that does not sound like altruism or an idealist's vision of a borderless global community of scientists working in harmony toward a common prize to be shared by all. If the above statement is surprising, consider the remarks of Congressman Ralph M. Hall of Texas, who opened hearings before the U.S. House of Representatives Subcommittee Scientific Cooperation as chairperson on October 19, 1989. Representative Hall admitted that the effort to map the genome would require the efforts of the international scientific community. He pointed out that given the magnitude of the project and the benefits to the whole world from having a blueprint of the human genetic structure, the question becomes "how does this country make sure that the basic research effort to map the human genome is shared equitably among its international scientific partners?" He stressed that "the nation who leads the applications resulting from the genome map will have a competitive advantage in pharmaceutical biotechnology and related issues."

James Watson who testified (sometimes testily) at the same hearing took the position that "it seems to me to make sense to try to reduce the final cost of the American public by having some form of sharing . . . we are paying a very large fraction of the bill and we want it to be clear from the very beginning that we are really not paying more than our fair share."

Watson, indulging in a bit of American chauvinism, said further, "we do a lot of work with them [the Japanese] but we don't need them. I think it should be clear." Earlier that month Watson had evoked an audible gasp from his audience when, speaking of Japan's alleged foot-dragging in their genome work and contributions to HUGO, he declared "I'm all for peace but if there is going to be a war, I will fight it."

While the redoubtable Watson was being characteristically feisty and many scientists had felt that he had gone too far in his vehemence, his call for financial as well as intellectual cooperation struck a resonant note with Congress. Times had changed from only two years earlier when Japan was feared as a tough competitor in the race to sequence the human genome. The prediction in 1987 that Japan was planning on achieving a 1 million base sequencing capability had been considerably scaled down to a goal of 100,000 bases per day and the Japanese initiative remains fragmented among four agencies.

The Japanese, understandably offended, responded in the words of Itaru Watanabe, vice president of the Science Council of Japan, that the HGP is not something that they are required to participate in "simply because the U.S. Government had decided to initiate and allocate a budget for it." Actually, the HGP is not alone in expecting foreign financial assistance. The National Academy of Sciences is putting pressure on Japanese industry to pay American colleges $100 million a year to narrow a "trading gap" produced by the presence of 24,000 Japanese students studying here. The DOE, in carrying out the goal of the Bush administration to pay for one third of the SSC with nonfederal funds, asked Japan and South Korea to come up with as much as $2.6 billion.

This request was based on a long tradition of international scientific cooperation among particle physicists in the building and running of each other's accelerators.

We are operating on two levels here. Scientists, like scholars in other disciplines, are accustomed to international cooperation, collaboration, and exchange of ideas and information. As a scientist the author can personally attest to the typical openness that has existed in this regard. But for the governments that support this research, the HGP is, in addition to its scientific merits, just another contributor in the arena of international competition. Is it possible to blend competitiveness with simultaneous cooperation? The Human Genome Organization (HUGO) hopes to do just that.

HUGO is loosely modeled on the European Molecular Biology Organization (EMBO), a consortium of 17 member nations formed to strengthen the training of European molecular biologists. While EMBO does not directly support research, it supports fellowships, scientific meetings, an excellent journal, workshops, and training courses. The founders of HUGO envisioned it as an international council to promote collaboration on the mapping and sequencing of the human genome. It is an extragovernmental organization with three major functions. The first is to facilitate discussion, dialogue, and coordination from scientists from around the world, particularly as regards the exchange of samples and technology. The second is the difficult process of trying to develop a means of collating and making readily available the mountains of data generated by the mapping and sequencing efforts of widely scattered groups who are using a variety of methods. Finally, the organization sponsors public debate and furnishes information on the scientific, legal, ethical, societal, and commercial applications of the HGP.

The membership, which numbered over 350 from more than 23 countries by 1991, is selected on the basis of merit in genome research. Walter Bodmer, director of research at the Imperial Cancer Research Fund in Britain, was elected to serve as HUGO president from 1990–1993, replacing Victor McCusick of Johns Hopkins University. Charles Cantor serves as the vice president for North America. Strapped for funds during the first two years of its existence, HUGO was given a strong boost in May 1990 by a $1 million four-year grant from the Howard Hughes Medical Institute. Earlier in 1990, the Wellcome Trust in the

U.K. announced a three-year grant for HUGO which provided $380,000 in the first year. The Wellcome trust derives its income mainly from Wellcome PC, an international pharmaceutical enterprise which operates in North America as Burroughs Wellcome.

George Cahill of HHMI, treasurer of HUGO, in contrast to what he calls Watson's "play(ing) hardball," favors "a more soft and more diplomatic" approach to encouraging international efforts. Walter Bodmer also points out that James Watson is not an active council member and his views are not necessarily those of HUGO. Bodmer regards as unenforceable restrictions on access to data suggested by Watson as a "punishment" for nations not contributing their fair share.

Perhaps "speaking softly" will be more effective in fulfilling HUGO's intended role, but do they "carry a big stick?" Certainly their membership is drawn from the power structure of the international genome scene. Among the HUGO council's 18 members, five are the leaders in the U.K. effort and five are from the U.S., two of whom (Leroy Hood and Victor McCusick) are also members of the Advisory Committee to the Center on Human Genome Research of the NIH.

However, as the "U.N. for the Human Genome Program," as Norton Zinder has aptly named it, HUGO's future as the self-appointed international arbiter and central clearinghouse for human genome analysis is by no means answered.

The United Nations, founded on the ideals of a peaceful world order, has been plagued with wars and other conflicts arising from national self-interest. HUGO, and in fact the entire HGP, faces in principle the same prospect. As we have pointed out, the HGP is a unique blend of scientific idealism operating in a framework of personal, corporate, and national competition.

DATA SHARING

The idealism is a reflection of the several levels on which the molecular genetics research of the HGP operates. The information generated by this kind of research may have commercial value, for example, in development of disease diagnostic tests or the isolation of a gene that can be put into a bacterial or yeast cell to make useful proteins. New procedures or instrumentation developed in the process may be patentable. Considerations other than free exchange of information enter into the public release of one's data when the issue of proprietary rights is involved.

The HGP in this regard is only part of a continuum that began with the advent of biotechnology in the late 1970s. The profit motive and the scientists searching for "truth" have come together in varying degrees of compatibility for over a decade with many questions still unanswered.

The "ideal" situation has been stated in various ways. James Watson, writing in 1990, hoped that "optimally, soon after new sequences are established, they will be added to a data base that is accessible world wide. . . . Making the sequence widely available as rapidly as practical is the only way to ensure that their full value will be realized and is the only acceptable way to handle information produced at public expense." Speaking at Human Genome II, Watson said that it is "hazy . . . whether people will hold onto important sequences." Charles Cantor, also at Human Genome II, warned that "if everybody hoards their little bit—then everything falls apart."

Walter Bodmer added on the same subject, "if we don't do it in an organized way we do it much less efficiently and costing much more money and if we do it on a collaborative basis then we provide the information . . . that we need to deal with the diseases that exist today." Later he admitted that "the problem is when new bits of DNA sequence are important there is bound to be lots of discussion on what to do with that—this is an area of very active study."

Since all participants in the HGP are studying the same subject, the human genome, it stands to reason that access to each other's findings would be helpful to at least avoid redundancy. Even more importantly this access would provide information that would be vital for what should be a large-scale collaborative effort. However, the U.S. government is supporting human genome research not only for the improvement of the nation's health but also as a national investment. Like the rest of biotechnology, this research is regarded as a source of direct and indirect economic benefits. Directly marketable products include such examples as DNA sequencers or DNA probes for diagnostic tests. Products such as maps and data bases which have no direct economic value will accelerate the development of products based on their use. All this is looked at as increasing our competitiveness at a time of increasing international trade imbalances and rising deficits. In this context, scientific inquiry is not considered out of the realm of trade.

This means that the government encourages the conversion of scientific knowledge into useful products, a process known as "technology transfer." Two of the goals listed in the DOE/NIH five-year plan (in the author's opinion itself an unfortunate term redolent of failed Communist Party agricultural programs) are to "enhance the already close working relationship with industry" and "encourage and facilitate the transfer of technologies and medically important information to the medical community." This will be done by a variety of approaches from direct federal funding of research at private companies to accelerating transfer of new molecular genetics technology into the private sector. Industry, in particular the pharmaceutical industry, will benefit by being able to hire scientists trained by the HGP and by drawing from the data generated by the HGP.

The Federal Technology Transfer Act of 1986 revised patent policies that pertained to federal labs. It literally mandated federal agencies like NIH to undertake industrial partnerships in order to encourage the transfer of technology as a means of increasing our international competitiveness. The act specifies that researchers are entitled to a minimum share of 15% of the royalties that may accrue from their work.

Those who oppose private ownership of genetic information feel that such ownership impedes access to data that have traditionally been published for general use. Will important steps in mapping and sequencing genetic material for diseases, for example, be held in secrecy until all of the details are worked out by the individual or the company involved? Would results published as they occurred enhance the chances of life-saving discoveries sooner?

University scientists need funding in order to carry on their work. This funding is granted based on their demonstrated expertise as well as the scientific merit of their proposed research as described in the grant application. It is therefore to the advantage of that scientist to publish results in a journal as soon as possible. This publication not only serves to enhance one's professional reputation but protects against someone else who might be working on the same project publishing his or her results earlier and thus being credited with the discovery. Scientists in private industry work in a different milieu. Their research, if it results in anything of proprietary value, must be kept "in house" until the required steps are taken to secure legal rights to the information.

However, few purists exist today. Collaboration with industry is very common among university-based researchers. The NIH found out how close this collaboration had become after it issued proposed guidelines on September 15, 1989. These were expected to eliminate potential conflicts of interest by government-funded university scientists who carried out clinical trials but they extended to nearly every segment of the biomedical community. Over the next several months NIH received about 800 letters of protest from scientists, professional societies, administrators, and biotech executives. The guidelines would have banned anyone receiving a research grant from having any financial ties to companies with links to the research being conducted, as well as forbidding any discussions of preliminary results with any such a company. It required full disclosure of all financial interests of scientists and their families, reviewers, and anyone else in a position to influence the research.

The overwhelming response to the proposal prompted Health and Human Services Secretary Louis Sullivan, to withdraw it. He told NIH officials to start again using an approach that stressed the value of the ties between university scientists and private industry. Sullivan asked for "new options . . . while keeping the research process free of unnecessary burdens and disincentives." He appeared to be affirming the position that the National Science Foundation (NSF) had made in its 14-page critique of the proposed guidelines that suggested that the proposed cure would be worse than the ailment. "After all," it pointed out, "in most cases the public can only benefit from research if some firm exploits the results commercially."

Despite fears by some that close ties with industry will tend to emphasize quick development and application of technology to the detriment of broad basic research, such collaboration is here to stay. In 1983 the then Health and Human Services Secretary, Margaret Heckler, declared, "NIH is an island of objective and pristine scientific research excellence untainted by commercialization influences." By mid-1990 NIH had developed about 200 close collaborations with business. But, for example, withholding information on the chromosomal location of a gene or on the sequence of a particularly interesting DNA segment until the rights to all the commercial applications flowing from that knowledge have been secured might be a natural reaction for a private company. Ironically, the leadership of the HGP can only hope that the exchange of information and cooperation needed to achieve their announced goals will not be unwittingly inhibited by a separate agenda driven by the profit motive.

*   *   *

We have briefly recounted the growing battles going on within the scientific community over whether or not the HGP as a bureaucratic entity is the maximally effective way to analyze the human genome. The fact remains that even if its demise might, at least according to some, slow the pace of such analysis, the (gene)ie is out of the bottle. Scientists will continue, in this country and elsewhere, to learn more and more about the precise chromosomal location and function of our genes. The potential for learning about the inner workings of living systems, coupled with the immediate possibilities of diagnosing and perhaps preventing and treating genetic disease, render impractical any thought of turning back from these goals.

In their pursuit, the opportunities and pressures to use this information will continue to grow. Some of these potential uses raise serious and troubling questions. The fair use of genetic information in employment and insurance, the dangers of infringement on personal privacy, the growing list of prenatal diagnostic capabilities, and other related issues need to be examined carefully.

Who will offer answers to these questions and on whose authority? We leave the world of science and enter that of ethics, always a necessary journey when science, morally neutral in its objective of attaining knowledge, uncovers secrets which can be used for good or ill.

11

GENES AND JUDGMENTS

The term "ethics" is used often but is much less frequently defined. According to *The American Heritage Dictionary*, ethics is "the study of the general nature of morals and of the specific moral choices to be made by the individual in his relationship with others; the philosophy of morals . . . the moral sciences as a whole including moral philosophy and customary civil and religious law." The term "moral" is defined as "of or concerned with the judgment of the goodness or badness of human action . . . pertaining to the discernment of good and evil."

Given these definitions, one can immediately understand why controversies over ethical questions can be so tortuous and protracted. Ethical choices demand decisions on moral questions. We can usually agree on general moral principles—the right of a person to his or her privacy or human dignity, for example. When we leave generalities and are faced with the complexities of weighing conflicting rights and obligations, the real debate begins.

Does an employer have a right to genetic information about an employee? Does an individual have a right to terminate the life of a human embryo or fetus? Can people be tested for a particular genetic disorder without their knowledge or against their will? Does a person have an obligation not to pass on disease-causing genes to his or her child? Am I obliged to share genetic information about myself with others, for example, my spouse, colleagues, the local blood bank, judge, insurance agent? Moreover, as so often happens in the case of human genetics and reproduction, some of these decisions must be translated into law.

It is obvious from these questions that morality and legality, while not synonymous, often share common ground. They intertwine and may be in one instance identical and in another at odds. The familiar objection that "you cannot legislate morality" is incorrect. Law is often an expression of society's moral values. For instance, whether established by authority, society, or custom, laws reflect a decision on what is acceptable and unacceptable behavior.

In the abortion controversy, quite relevant to this chapter, there are those who maintain that despite the legality of abortion it is immoral to terminate the life of a human embryo or fetus. They argue that the law should be changed to reflect that moral judgment. Opponents argue that since there is disagreement about the morality of such an act, individuals ought to be free to make such a decision in private.

In creating laws we are often faced with defining moral values that guide human behavior. It seems logical to some to assume that such decisions need to be made relative to a set of basic principles. For example, Edmond Pellegrino, director of the Center for the Advanced Study of Ethics at Georgetown University, responded to our request for a statement on this problem. He replied that

> resolution of the major issues arising from the Human Genome Project is sure to be enormously complicated by the lack of a coherent philosophy of human nature in contemporary philosophy. Without such a philosophy ethical norms cannot be grounded and there is little likelihood of agreement upon the limits between licit and illicit uses of genetic information and technology. Without a coherent view of the nature and purposes of human existence—individual and communal—ethics must fall back into libertarian individualism and consensual ethics—the pragmatic resolution of ethical conflict by legal and political processes. Perhaps more than any other biotechnological advance genetic mapping uncovers the moral poverty of current trends which reduce philosophy to a handmaiden of science and ethics to political consensus. Like atomic power, genetics can free or enslave. Only through monitoring by a rigorous ethic grounded in some objective standard of morality can genetics become the instrument of individual and social good.

Pellegrino's statement, which is representative of a widely held school of thought, appears to leave little hope for an easy resolution to the ethical dilemmas that are presented to us by the study of human genetics.

If genetics can become an "instrument of individual and social good" only through a "rigorous ethic grounded in some objective standard of morality," what is the alternative if such a standard is unavailable or at least not agreed upon?

There are those who take a position on ethics quite the opposite of Pellegrino's. Santiago Grisolia, director of the Cell Research Institute and Distinguished Professor of Biochemistry at the University of Kansas Medical School, writes in *Hastings Center Report* that "Science is, or at least should be, based on objectivity. And therein lies its conflict with ethics, because ethics as such is not an objective discipline. Rather, it tends more to employ principles that vary with time and people."

C. Keith Boone, associate dean of the College of Arts and Sciences at Denison University, states in that same journal that "no ethical tradition seems sufficient to comprehend either the peculiarity of the genetic dilemma or the multiplicity of moral conundrums it presents."

If, as George Annas claims in the *Hastings Center Report*, it is true that "we are utterly unprepared to deal with issues of mandatory [genetic] screening, confidentiality, privacy, and discrimination," we still have no choice but to confront these issues in the problematic arena of our pluralistic society.

Our intention here is first to summarize both the current state of and anticipated advances in knowledge about the human genome, specifically in relation to disease. Second, the rapid advances in the understanding of our genome have brought increased attention and urgency to ethical issues with which society has wrestled for a long time and which, according to some, have raised new critical questions as well. We will outline what these issues are in the context of diagnosis of genetic disease or predisposition to genetic disease in both the prenatal and postnatal context. Third, we will point out major social implications of these issues in such areas as medical care, employment, and insurance.

Finally, the efforts of the NIH National Center for Human Genome Research and the DOE Human Genome Program to address these issues will be described. The NIH has declared its ongoing commitment to "support activities that focus on anticipating issues arising from the application of the results of the Human Genome Initiative and on proposing solutions that will forestall adverse effects." They have taken on a daunting challenge.

MEDICAL GENETICS

Medical genetics deals with the diagnosis, treatment, causes, and prevention of disorders linked to genes. There are four types of such disorders: (1) single gene, (2) multiple genes, (3) gross chromosome abnormalities, and (4) genetic damage due to exposure to harmful environmental agents.

1. Single gene. All of us harbor potentially harmful genes in our chromosomes. These are usually "recessive" genes and as such they do not cause harm unless they combine with another recessive gene during sexual reproduction. If two "carriers," people who carry the same recessive gene, reproduce, the chances are one in four that both of the genes, and thus the disease, will be passed on to the child. Examples of such single-gene disorders are cystic fibrosis, sickle-cell anemia, and retinoblastoma (a retinal cancer in children.)

Sometimes the harmful genes are dominant. In this case the parent who has the dominant gene will also have the disorder. There is a 50% chance that the gene will be passed on to the child. Examples are Huntington's disease, neurofibromatosis (nerve tumors), and hyper-cholesterolemia (excessive amounts of cholesterol in the blood).

Moreover, a disease-causing recessive gene may be located on the X chromosome. It will then be expressed in the male, who is XY, but not in the female, who is XX, except in the rare instance when the gene is found on both X chromosomes. Prominent examples are hemophilia and Du-chenne muscular dystrophy.

2. Multiple genes—also called polygenic. Multiple genes with their additive effects cause many disorders. Some of these are cleft palate, club foot, diabetes mellitus, urinary tract malfunctions, and spina bifida. Since an as yet unspecified number of genes contribute to these disorders, the chances of inheriting such conditions are not as readily predictable as others such as cystic fibrosis.

3. Gross chromosome abnormalities. There may be too few or too many chromosomes, or a chromosome may be damaged. Most such abnormalities cause death to the embryo. Some survive, however. For example, individuals with an extra chromosome number 21 have Down's syndrome characterized by mental retardation.

4. Exposure to harmful environmental agents. Such exposure can damage genes at any stage of life. For example, viral infections such as German measles (rubella) or HIV (AIDS) during pregnancy may cause a variety of developmental defects in the child. Abuse of alcohol during pregnancy may result in fetal alcohol syndrome, characterized by brain damage and facial deformity. Currently there are over 50 genetic diseases that can increase a person's susceptibility to toxic or cancerous effects of environmental agents. This is of particular significance in genetic testing of employees who might be exposed to such conditions.

In 1976 the National Genetic Disease Act provided federal support for a national genetic disease testing, counseling, and education program. There are now many such genetic services, both public and private, available nationwide. Networks of genetics service providers have been established who coordinate research and education with each region of the United States Department of Health and Human Services. Until recently, tests for genetic disorders were not based on direct DNA analysis. They depended on, for example, taking family histories to determine the familial incidence of inherited disorders. This sometimes could enable one to calculate the odds of a disorder occurring in a child planned by a couple seeking advice. If a woman was already pregnant, another common practice has been studying fetal cells for chromosome numbers or assaying for abnormal fetal gene products in order to detect the presence of an abnormality.

The latter approach has been used to determine carriers as well, such as in the case of Tay–Sachs disease, a tragic condition in which the nervous system degenerates. This most commonly occurs among Jews of Eastern European descent. Within this population it strikes one child in 3600 and the child usually dies before the age of 4. The reduced activity of a particular enzyme in an adult indicates that he or she carries the Tay–Sachs gene. Also, in prenatal diagnosis of this condition, the absence of the enzyme product indicates that the fetus has the disease.

Our particular interest here are those genes whose presence can be detected, not by looking for gene products or gross chromosome abnormalities, but for the genes themselves. Only approximately 100 genes involved in the more than 3000 known heritable diseases have been isolated. The HGP will rapidly add to this number.

DNA can be isolated easily from almost any cells of the body. Even cells rinsed from the lining of the mouth provide enough DNA for gene characterization. The revolutionary polymerase chain reaction (PCR), which we described in Chapter 7, permits the amplification of a minuscule sample of DNA into quantities sufficient for molecular analytical techniques. DNA can be stored indefinitely, so that samples from individuals with genetic problems can be used later to help diagnose other family members.

Once in hand, the DNA can be analyzed using techniques also described previously in Chapter 6, that is, RFLPs or specific DNA probes. To summarize these briefly, naturally occurring variations among individuals in the nitrogenous base sequences of their DNA result in differing lengths of DNA when it is cut up into pieces by restriction enzymes. The differences in base sequences are referred to as restriction length polymorphism (RFLP) markers.

The restriction enzymes cut DNA at specific sites marked by a particular series of nitrogenous bases. If this cutting site happens to be located near a particular disease gene, that gene will be nearly always associated with the fragment produced by the action of the restriction enzyme. Even when a disease gene has not been identified or its exact location is not known, the presence of the RFLP fragment can be used as an indication that the gene is present.

The pattern of RFLP marker inheritance within a family can be followed and the inheritance pattern used to pinpoint the inheritance of the disease gene. One of the first dramatic instances of the successful application of this technology was in 1983 when the linkage between an RFLP on chromosome number 4 and Huntington's disease was described.

RFLP analysis is useful within families when the exact nature of the gene is not known but its presence can be discerned by examining patterns of RFLP inheritance. This indirect form of gene detection is often used in prenatal diagnosis but is also useful for some adult conditions such as polycystic kidney disease (APKD). This condition is characterized by the slow growth of cysts in the kidneys, usually beginning between the ages of 20 to 35. This growth ultimately destroys the kidneys. Several RFLP markers have been found very close to the

APKD site on chromosome number 16. RFLP analysis of affected and unaffected family members may allow prediction of the onset of this disease long before symptoms occur.

The study of RFLP markers has shown linkages to a number of single-gene diseases such as Duchenne muscular dystrophy (progressive muscle deterioration), phenylketonuria (lack of an enzyme that causes brain damage and mental retardation), and retinoblastoma (cancer of the eye). As the number of available RFLP markers increases through the HGP, the number of genetic diseases that can be diagnosed will likewise increase.

In a few cases genes responsible for disease can be directly detected using restriction enzymes followed by using specific DNA probes which are either the actual genes, parts of genes, or synthetic DNA sequences. Once a gene is sequenced a probe can be made in the lab that will recognize and bind to the gene in question. This method is used to detect the sickle-cell gene, hemophilia (type A), and cystic fibrosis. A complete physical map of the human genome, another goal of the HGP, will eventually be the ultimate source of DNA probes for any human gene.

Currently, only a handful of tests are commercially available that can be used to identify genes which diagnose the presence of a disease. Scientists expect that this number will rapidly expand along with the number of markers. That will lead to a situation that raises even tougher questions—the identity of those at risk of future disease.

PREDICTIVE MEDICINE

Here we are no longer talking about diagnosing an individual as a carrier or as one who has a symptomatic disease. We are looking at the detection of a gene or group of genes whose presence predicts various levels of risk for future illness. The report of such genetic analysis would not be expressed as "this individual is a carrier of disease A or has disease A," but "this individual at some time in the future will or is likely to develop disease A." Medicine in this case becomes predictive, and if possible, preventive.

Prominent among the possibilities are some of the leading causes of human death: cancer and cardiovascular disease or others such as emphysema, diabetes, and mental illness. Each of these presents a complex scientific puzzle because the expression of these disorders often includes a genetic component. This in turn interacts with various environmental factors such as diet and stress.

Cardiovascular Disease

About 20 genes regulate the level of cholesterol in the blood. The differing nature and function of this polygenic complex among individuals puts some at greater risk of early coronary artery disease and heart attacks. Several mutations have been identified in one of those genes that are sufficient to cause premature onset of one form of arteriosclerosis (hardening of the arteries). The genetic defect leads to a buildup of low-density lipoproteins (LDL)—a complex of cholesterol and protein that is deposited on the lining of the blood vessels and can lead to heart attacks before the age of 40. Tests have shown that about 1 in 500 persons carries the mutant gene.

Diabetes

Millions currently suffer from this abnormality in which, in certain types of diabetes, cells in the immune system suddenly attack and destroy the insulin-making cells in the pancreas. Sugar metabolism is affected and survival is possible only with careful monitoring of diet and regular doses of insulin. A gene mutation in DNA taken from white blood cells first detected in 1989 may lead to the identification of individuals who have inherited the tendency to develop this serious disease. Amazingly, five research groups virtually simultaneously isolated the gene for a protein, known as a glucose transporter, that appears to be crucial in the normal movement of glucose (blood sugar) from the blood into the body's cells. Perhaps an inborn defect in this transporter predisposes some individuals to the disease.

Cancer

Since 1983 scientists have found over 50 "oncogenes," genes associated with various forms of cancers. The genes are needed for normal growth but can switch over to stimulate tumor production by a variety of mostly as-yet-unspecified environmental factors. Five million persons now have cancer, which has turned out to be a very complex genetic disease. The exact link between a particular gene and a specific type of tumor is still unclear. Cancers appear to be triggered by multiple gene problems. For example, up to ten mutations in various genes may need to occur in colon cells before cancer begins. There are now some tests available to detect some of these premalignant changes. The discovery could possibly identify individuals at risk for cancer even before it develops.

In 1990, researchers at the Massachusetts General Hospital Cancer Center reported that in the rare Li–Fraumeni syndrome, in which children are born with an identifiable damaged form of a cancer-suppressing gene, the children often develop a variety of cancers including brain tumors, breast cancer, and bone cancer at an early age. Scientists predict that other forms of the inherited mutant gene probably causing other cancers that show up in families will be identified.

Mental Illness

Alzheimer's disease, manic-depressive illness, and schizophrenia, which together afflict 4 million people, have all been shown to have genetic components. Alzheimer's, a degeneration of the central nervous system characterized by memory impairment and diminished intellectual function beginning in middle to late adulthood, progresses to a profound mental and physical disability that eventually necessitates institutional care. One form of Alzheimer's representing about 10% of the known cases appears to be caused by a genetic defect on chromosome 21.

In a study of the Old Order Amish community of southeastern Pennsylvania, a gene located on chromosome 11 was reported in 1987 to be active in manic-depressive illness. This tragic condition is referred to as a bipolar disorder because of the person's severe mood swings, which oscillate between deep depression and euphoria. Those who inherit the gene have about a 60% chance of developing the disease as an adult.

Other scientists searching along the length of chromosome 11 from non-Amish families did not find the same gene. But soon afterward yet another manic-depressive gene was located on the X chromosome of still other families. Once again, we have a situation where genes are influential but other as yet unknown elements are at work.

PRENATAL TESTING

In reproduction, one of the millions of tiny human sperm cells swarming about the relatively massive egg in the upper reaches of the oviduct gains entrance through the egg membrane. The 23 chromosomes that the sperm carries as a genetic legacy from the father line up next to the 23 maternal chromosomes in the egg. If all goes well, these 46 strands of DNA, now a totally unique combination of genes, will begin to respond to cues as yet unknown to science and begin the complex dance of replication and separation known as cell division.

The fertilized egg, now referred to as the "embryo," becomes two cells, then four cells, and so on. At each stage the enclosed genes somehow are signaled to become active or to remain dormant, awaiting their turn. The embryo grows in size and complexity. By eight weeks after fertilization, long since buried in the protective warm tissue lining the uterus, it has shaped itself into a miniature human organism. So immediately recognizable as human, though still minute, it is now called a "fetus" or literally "the offspring."

It is a hazardous journey from egg to fetus. Before highly sensitive hormonal methods for early detection of pregnancy were available, the frequency of miscarriage anytime after fertilization was considered to be about 15%. We now think that perhaps as many as 80% of human fertilized eggs do not survive. They succumb silently and undetected.

Hidden in the womb, the embryo or fetus cannot be examined

directly. But as the fetus grows it is surrounded by a protective pool of fluid. It sheds cells into this "amniotic" fluid. Sampling was for a long time possible only by the 16th week of pregnancy in a process known as "amniocentesis." This was and is accomplished by inserting a long needle into the fluid-filled sac housing the fetus. First used to predict the need for blood transfusions for the newborn when an RH factor incompatibility was suspected, amniocentesis was later employed to prepare a karyotype. This is a preparation of chromosomes spread out on a slide and stained. The slide can then be examined through a microscope to determine the sex or any gross chromosomal abnormalities that might be present.

Once this technology was in place, dozens of biochemical tests were developed to uncover metabolic defects. These defects ranged from relatively harmless to devastating disabilities such as Tay–Sachs disease.

"Alpha fetoprotein," which can be detected also in the blood of the pregnant woman, is a substance that diffuses from the fetus because of the failure of the vertebrae to completely close over the spinal cord. Its presence can mean disorders in the fetus, such as anencephaly, in which major parts of the brain do not develop, or spina bifida, which ranges from a mild condition to one in which paralysis or even death can result.

By growing fetal cells in the laboratory and using PCR to copy the cells' DNA, the fetal genome can be analyzed in as much detail as DNA from any other source. And rather than have to wait until four months of pregnancy have passed, using a procedure called chorionic villus biopsy, physicians can now insert a thin sterile device up into the uterus by eight weeks after fertilization and snip out a tiny piece of the young placenta. This tissue is made entirely of cells from the embryo. A minute sample is all that is needed to feed to the PCR apparatus in which the DNA is cloned for analysis.

There is now no known treatment or cure for the vast majority of genetic disorders which can be diagnosed. It is probably unrealistic to expect that many such cures or treatments will be developed in the near future. We can predict with some certainty, however, that the list of identifiable genetic disorders will grow rapidly. We are left in the paradoxical position of diagnosing and predicting the onset of many genetic and gene-influenced diseases from which there is no escape. That is, unless the analysis is done before birth.

ABORTION

There is perhaps no more contentious issue in our society than the issue of abortion. Widely disparate views are argued with equal fervor among physicians, clergy, feminists, sociologists, and everyone else who possess a set of convictions or are invited to express them—which leaves out very few of us.

Ever since the landmark *Roe v. Wade* Supreme Court decision in 1973 elective abortion has been legal in this country. In 1989 there were approximately 1,500,000 abortions performed in the United States. Despite the many protests lodged against this decision it has remained in effect and will more than likely continue to be allowed unless a strong political consensus develops to reverse it. We can proceed, therefore, with the assumption that abortion is and will continue to be an available legal option.

Genetic disorders occur in about 4% of all live births while gross chromosomal defects are seen in another 0.5%. Altogether they account for about one quarter of all U.S. pediatric hospital admissions and 12% of all the adult admissions in this country. Behind the percentages are some arresting annual numbers—6000 to 8000 cases of spina bifida, 5000 children with Down's syndrome, 1500 with cystic fibrosis and over 1000 newborns with sickle-cell anemia. The incidence of fetal chromosome abnormalities increases as women age. The risk in a pregnancy for a 20-year-old woman is 1 in 526. By age 38 it is 1 in 102, and by 45 it rises to 1 in 21.

Although the legal right to abort precludes one from having to qualify for such a procedure by offering proof that the embryo or fetus is seriously impaired, no one would deny that there is a spectrum of severity of genetic conditions which can be uncovered by prenatal testing. The extremes of the spectrum are clear. On one hand, a woman may decide to abort after a karyotype reveals the sex of the fetus. On the other hand, a diagnosis of Tay–Sachs, for example, poses a very different set of circumstances on which to base an abortion decision.

In both cases the woman has a legal right to her decision but the reasons informing her choice are quite distinct. A woman is faced with a different complex of considerations depending on the nature of the genetic condition diagnosed. Suppose that Down's syndrome is the prenatal diagnosis. The child will survive but will be mentally retarded. The degree of severity cannot be predicted. For example, the author's sister has Down's syndrome, can read and write, and for many years was a comforting companion to her parents. Conversely, other parents will feel unable to cope with the special needs of a child with Down's. Approximately 35% of Down's children have congenital heart disease which leads to their death, usually by the fourth or fifth decade of life. Also, many develop Alzheimer's disease.

And what of cystic fibrosis? The discovery of the cystic fibrosis gene in 1989 has allowed testing for the presence of the gene in both children, adults, and prenatally. However, as we have pointed out, the existing test is imperfect. Because of the number of possible mutations in the gene it permits an unequivocal diagnosis of carriers in only about half the cases (the rest will not be detected)—and the prenatal test which detects the presence of a mutant gene that will cause cystic fibrosis does not predict the severity of the condition.

In March 1990, the American Society of Human Genetics and the NIH issued guidelines advising against mass testing for the gene until the detection rate of 95% could be achieved. They called for pilot studies on how best to carry out a testing program. Despite the possibility of diagnosing this most common fatal genetic disorder among Caucasians, a year and a half after the gene's discovery financial support for a pilot program was not available.

Robert Beall, executive vice president and medical director at the Cystic Fibrosis Foundation, an organization whose mission is to find a treatment and cure for this disease, explained in *Science* the foundation's decision not to fund a screening study: "For us to invest in issues outside our major mission," said Beall, "would take funds away from the work we do."

The *Science* report goes on to say that sources close to foundation officials say that the abortion controversy played a role in that decision. There was reportedly a fear that "by supporting screening—and thus, implicitly, abortion of affected fetuses—they would risk losing the financial contributions that make their research possible."

If both parents are definitely diagnosed as cystic fibrosis carriers, they cannot be sure that a negative prenatal test is accurate. In addition, recent experiments have shown some promise toward an eventual treatment for cystic fibrosis. While this raises the hopes of parents with children suffering from cystic fibrosis it makes a prenatal decision even more difficult. Added to the equation now is the scenario of a future treatment or even a cure through gene therapy.

Equally problematic in this regard is the prenatal diagnosis of Huntington's disease. Here we are looking at finding a dominant gene that will invariably trigger an ultimately fatal degenerative disease perhaps 40 or 50 years later. It also means, of course, that at least one of the parents who has the gene will eventually develop the symptoms. The use of RFLP markers requires the testing of other family members, at least one of whom must be known to have the disease. The grandparent with the disease gene may or may not pass it on to the prospective parent—a positive fetal test will indicate that this had occurred. If one parent has the gene, the odds of transmitting it in a future pregnancy is 50%.

Should a couple be encouraged by the advances in molecular genetics that led to locating the approximate chromosomal placement of the Huntington's gene? Will scientists eventually be able to isolate it? Should they put their faith in the development of a cure for the disease before their child becomes symptomatic?

A potentially even more bewildering set of circumstances arises when medical genetics predicts not necessarily the certainty but the increased likelihood of the onset of a disease later in life, perhaps not even until adulthood.

This "predictive diagnosis" causes even more ambivalence when we consider the variety of genetic predictions that already are becoming available. A genetic profile can reveal a variety of possible predispositions from alcoholism to heart disease to manic-depression to schizo-phrenia. This kind of partial knowledge complicates matters even further.

Of course, in theory, as diagnoses for both single-gene and poly-genic disorders are perfected, a gene profile for every fetus will reveal several genes responsible for the ills to which all humans are heir. We are now in only the early transition to that era.

Strictly in terms of genetics, it might seem that prenatal diagnosis and selective abortion would eventually eliminate altogether the genes responsible for disease. Even looked at in this impersonal way in some cases this would have precisely the opposite effect. A couple who already had a child with Tay–Sachs or cystic fibrosis or who were both diagnosed as being carriers for these diseases could elect to have no children. In that case they would not pass on their recessive genes to the next generation and their genes would be removed from the population. But if they successively aborted fetuses who had inherited both recessive genes until giving birth to a normal child, this offspring would have a 50–50 chance of being a carrier. Thus the genes would survive.

What is one to do in the face of prenatal diagnosis expressed in terms of statistical probabilities, as a prediction of an illness far in the future, or even a predisposition to physical or mental disorders to which millions of people are prone?

Given the array of genetic problems that can now be found or predicted and the certainty that many more will be added to the list, the decision about whether or not to terminate a pregnancy is being colored by new questions. Since abortion is a free personal decision will the person making the free choice not to abort have to take on the respon-sibility for the consequences? That is, having knowingly given birth to a child whose medical care is extremely expensive will society continue to accept the cost? What of those whose personal or religious convictions do not allow them to consider abortion as a moral option? To deny access to care for a child with an inherited disease or to make that care prohib-itively expensive would be tantamount to offering the parents no choice at all.

John Hodgson, writing in *Trends in Biotechnology*, warned that "Responsible scientists active in human genetics . . . must aim to insure that society can say to the patient in effect, 'It's up to you to choose and we will support you in either choice.' " Who can predict with certainty that society will be so benign? In the early 1970s several states passed laws (since repealed or unenforced) that required sickle-cell carrier tests for a marriage license or school attendance. In 1989 a bill was introduced into the Texas legislature which would have made it a crime for a woman infected with the AIDs virus to bear a child.

The bill did not pass, but will the rationale behind it permit others to legislate against bearing genetically "defective children"? After all, the technology for diagnosis is available. Are women and their physicians to be required to use it? Would it be assumed that a positive prenatal diagnosis will be automatically followed by abortion?

In 1978 the New York State Court of Appeals ruled that parents could sue physicians for not warning them of their risks of predictable genetic disorders and further ruled that the physician could be financially responsible for the costs of caring for the child. In 1980 the California State Court of Appeals awarded damages to a baby with Tay–Sachs disease because she had "the right . . . to receive damages for the pain and suffering underwent during the limited life span available. . . . The certainty of genetic impairment is no longer a mystery." The court denied the parents' request for blaming the physician for "wrongful causation of life" because the child had been denied the "fundamental right of a child to be born as a wholly functional human being." The court held that "whether it is better to have been born at all than to have been born with gross deficiencies is a mystery more properly left to the philosophers and the theologians."

Granted, the vast majority of the abortions performed annually in the United States are not done because of an unfavorable prenatal diagnosis. But for those couples who do seek and obtain such a diagnosis will the freedom to abort move inexorably toward the status of an obligation?

Nancy Wexler, in her address at Human Genome II, warned against the fallacy of the "apocryphal body shoppers." She took the position that most women who opt for prenatal genetic testing "do not want a perfect baby." They "want one that will not rue the day it was born." Perhaps that is so, but will the power of genetic analysis bias our ideas not of what is perfect but what is normal? Is a child "abnormal" who may, under certain conditions, be somewhat more likely to develop cancer, manic-depression, or be of limited intelligence? What about the child who will never walk or have full control over his or her lower extremities but who might someday contribute brilliant ideas, art, or music to his or her society?

EUGENICS

In 1871 Charles Darwin, in *The Descent of Man*, stated that "the weak members of civilized society propagate their kind. No one who has attended to the breeding of domestic animals will doubt that this must be highly injurious to the race of man . . . hardly anyone is so ignorant as to allow his worst animals to breed."

Darwin's cousin, Frances Galton—a prominent British anthropologist—avidly supported this philosophy. He recommended its application in particular "to produce a highly gifted race of men by judicious marriages during several consecutive generations." He coined the term "eugenics" from the Greek "eugenes" meaning "endowed by heredity with noble qualities." Eugenics can be defined as "methods of improving the quality of the human race, especially by selective breeding."

As taught and practiced over the next 75 years, eugenics retained this notion of improving the human race by breeding "better" people. The major emphasis was on the inheritance of intelligence, ability, or virtue and the elimination of "feeblemindedness" or "depravity." It was based on almost total misunderstanding of the nature of human heredity. Its practitioners were ignorant of what is still a complex, poorly understood interplay among genes and between genes and the environment in which they act.

Ironically, the early eugenics movement in America was centered at Cold Spring Harbor, now headed by James Watson. Charles Davenport, professor at the University of Chicago, had returned home after having visited with Galton and others in England filled with "renewed courage for the fight for the quantitative study of evolution." He persuaded the Carnegie Institute of Washington to establish a station for that purpose at

Cold Spring Harbor where Davenport was already the director of a summer biological field station. He launched a major effort to gather family histories, assuming that race determined behavior. He identified the best human genetic endowment with that of the white middle class— intellectuals, musicians, artists, and, of course, scientists.

Galton had promoted "positive eugenics," the procreation between people of supposed good genetic endowment. Davenport's emphasis was on "negative eugenics"—the prevention of mating by people with supposed undesirable characteristics such as feeblemindedness—a catch-all for mental disorders which we now know are a complex and still little understood mix of genetic endowment and environmental influences.

In his popular 1911 book, *Heredity in Relation to Eugenics*, Davenport wrote that ". . . the rights of society over the life, the reproduction, the behavior, and the acts of the individuals that compose it are in all matters concerning the life and proper progress of society limitless and society may take life, may sterilize, may segregate so as to prevent marriage, may restrict liberty in a hundred ways."

The wide acceptance of this semiscientific teaching led inexorably to selective immigration policies and state-sponsored sterilization. According to Davenport, "The idea of a melting pot belongs to a pre-Mendelian age." By 1930, 24 states had laws on the books allowing sterilization of a wide variety of "undesirables"—epileptics, the "insane," or habitual criminals. In April 1924, the Immigration Act enforcing quotas on other nationalities was signed into law by President Calvin Coolidge. He had earlier declared "America must be kept American. . . . Biological laws show . . . that Nordics deteriorate when mixed with other races."

When Adolph Hitler advocated eugenic sterilization in 1923, his views were consistent with many reputable geneticists in Europe and North America. This was followed in 1933 by a "law on the prevention of hereditary disease in future generations." In 1934, 56,000 orders for sterilization were issued. After 1935, eugenic and racial policies merged. In 1939 the Third Reich went far beyond sterilization and marriage prohibition to the systematic killing of the mentally ill and of all Jews.

Even after the war, the notion of the acceptability of negative eugenics lingered. A popular textbook, *General Zoology*, whose fourth edition was published in 1965, stated "Eugenists seek to . . . encourage legislation that will prevent matings between obviously defective persons."

It is no wonder that the very word eugenics has now become a pejorative? It is also not surprising that modern geneticists are exquisitely sensitive to any public perception that their discipline is linked to any notion of a "master race." James Watson admitted that "the shadows of past abuses loom in the background of genetic research. We can prevent such atrocities from recurring if scientists, doctors, and society at large refuse to cede control of genetic discoveries to those who would misuse them."

George Annas, coauthor of *Reproductive Genetics and the Law*, lists as prominent among the ethical issues that could seriously interfere with the current support for the HGP the need for judiciously "resisting a eugenic agenda."

In January 1989, the European Parliament insisted that the human genome studies supported by the European Economic Community be open to public scrutiny so that they would not lead to "neo-eugenics." The original human genome program as proposed by the European commission aimed at identifying "high-risk individuals" in order to "protect them from illnesses to which they are most genetically vulnerable and where appropriate to prevent the transmission of genetic susceptibilities to the next generation." An editorial in *New Scientist* advised that "unless (the spectre of eugenics) is exorcized the ghost may well scare some Europeans out of doing the science."

Consequently, the commission rewrote its objections, deleting references to "predictive medicine" including medical risk forecasting or transferring genetic techniques to medicine. It called for a committee to oversee the program and conduct in-depth discussions of the ethical, social, and legal aspects of human genome analysis. The committee would be charged with identifying any "possible misuses."

GENETIC SCREENING

A growing list of tests using PCR, DNA probes, and RFLPs are now available that can diagnose genetic diseases. They can also identify

individuals as carriers of disease genes, pinpoint gene-based susceptibilities or predisposition to a wide variety of diseases, and in some cases
predict the eventual onset of disease long before symptoms occur.

Unfortunately, whether obtained pre- or postnatally, positive test
results, rather than indicating treatment modalities as is so often the case
in nongenetic disease, only serve to underline the growing gap between
diagnosis and treatment.

Carrier detection, when coupled with expert and effective counseling, can often clearly indicate the odds of transmitting genetic disease,
particularly when the chromosomes of both partners are analyzed.
Should this be a voluntary, private procedure as it is now practiced? Or
should it be a mass screening of a population, whether voluntary or
mandatory? Who should have access to the results?

The prevention of transmission of a genetic disease to the next
generation must be weighed against the danger of a social stigma being
placed on carriers resulting in, for example, discrimination in employment. The relative rights of individuals must be weighed against concerns of public health. Claims to the test results by third parties such as
employers, insurance companies, or relatives would have to be balanced
against the individual's right to privacy.

Serious problems have arisen when enthusiasm for implementing
genetic screening programs have outweighed caution because of lack of
experience in their safety and benefit. As far back as the early 1960s a
biochemical test for phenylketonuria (PKU) in newborns led to mandatory newborn screening in most states by 1967. This single-gene disorder, in which a missing enzyme prevents the breakdown of the amino
acid phenylalanine, leads to a toxic buildup of this chemical in the blood
with resulting brain damage.

Theoretically, a diet low in phenylalanine is the ideal treatment. In
the haste to set up screening programs a lack of experience in regulating
the diet, incorrect diagnoses, and subsequent treatment of children with
false positives led to a number of infant deaths. By the mid-1970s quality
controls were in place and mandatory PKU screening of newborns
continues to this day as an effective diagnostic tool.

Similarly, by 1972, after a simple and relatively reliable test for
sickle-cell anemia was developed, 12 states had passed legislation man-
dating sickle-cell screening of blacks without adequate provision for

patient or public education. For example, in Massachusetts, a sickle-cell test was requested for admission to school, and in New York it was required in order to obtain a marriage license. Misunderstanding the implications of the test led to discrimination in employment and life insurance.

The black community reacted by pushing for more research into the problem and for voluntary testing. The National Sickle-Cell Anemia Control Act of 1972 forbids funding for testing except for those states who have voluntary programs. The 1972 act was amended four years later to the National Sickle-Cell Anemia, Cooley's Anemia, Tay–Sachs and Genetic Disease Act. It mandated increased levels of basic and applied research, training, testing, counseling, and public education in sickle-cell anemia as well as other genetic diseases.

As recently as 1980 a black student sued the Air Force Academy alleging that he was unfairly denied entrance because the Academy's mandatory sickle-cell screening had shown that he was a sickle-cell carrier. It had been the practice at the Academy to automatically disqualify black applicants if they were carriers of the gene. There is still controversy over whether carriers of sickle-cell trait are at any risk under conditions of oxygen stress such as high altitude. A 1974 National Academy of Sciences report stated that "there was insufficient scientific information to form a basis for excluding carriers from the armed forces." In 1981, the Academy backed down and reversed their policy.

"An International Survey of Attitudes of Medical Geneticists towards Mass Screening Access to Results" was published in *Public Health Reports*. Six hundred seventy-seven medical geneticists in 18 countries responded to this survey which included a series of questions on mass screening for cystic fibrosis carriers. In the absence of absolute answers it is instructive to pay careful attention to the people who confront genetic problems on a daily basis.

The survey asked for opinions based on a theoretical availability of a cheap, accurate cystic fibrosis test. Seventy-five percent of the respondents felt that the most important objective of mass screening was informed reproductive choices for carriers and that CF screening at whatever age should be voluntary. Eighty-two percent thought that screening should be applied on a voluntary basis to the entire population.

There was no consensus about the optimal age for screening.

Thirteen percent would permit screening of children or adolescents younger than 18 with parental consent. Thirty-seven percent advocated screening adults over 18 by consent and 5% suggested screening several other ages by law.

A total of 78% gave greatest weight to the welfare of the person being screened, 10% to the welfare of society, and 9% to the health of future generations. Only 4% expressed concern over carrier discrimination, which surprised the authors of the survey in view of well-known experiences with mass sickle-cell screening.

The scene surrounding proposed mass screening for the cystic fibrosis gene is a useful paradigm for the debates which are sure to follow over screening for other genes. In 1989, several biotechnology companies announced plans to market screening services for cystic fibrosis. Concern arose that, left to free market forces, pressures to use the test would be felt by physicians because of fear of liability if the tests were available and not used. In the U.S. more than 8 million people are probably CF gene carriers. At $100 to $200 per test, even if only the 2.4 million couples who marry each year were tested, would fear and anxiety arouse such pressures that millions would demand screening? CF screening is a potential billion dollar industry.

Make no mistake about the commercial possibilities of genetic testing. Such technology is in its infancy but entrepreneurs are ready. Advertisements have already been published in reputable magazines announcing the availability of services which include the long-term storage of blood cells. These would be stored and made available for future use in genetic linkage analysis, which, as we have explained, requires DNA from individuals affected by a genetic disease as well as DNA from unaffected family members. At any time in the future, then, by analyzing the patterns of inheritance of genetic markers such as RFLPs linked closely to genes causing disease, conclusions can be drawn about which family members are at risk for the disease. While Grandpa may be deceased, his cells and their DNA will be stored for disease diagnosis of future generations.

According to Benjamin Wilfond and Norman Fost of the Department of Pediatrics and the program in medical ethics at the University of Wisconsin School of Medicine, "Mass genetic screening programs should be considered experimental public health programs implemented only after a favorable assessment of a program that effectively achieves its goal which minimizes the potential medical, ethical, legal and social problems."

They pointed out the criticizable elements of such a program not least of which is the danger of both false-positive and false-negative results. According to their calculations, in testing couples from families without a history of CF "one of every two couples from the general population who would be identified to be at risk would be falsely labeled." They urged that screening be limited to high-risk groups until the possibility of false positives is less than 0.1%.

Even assuming test accuracy, a critical consideration in genetic screening as well as genetic testing of any kind is the availability and quality of counseling. Here we are faced with widespread lack of understanding about genetic disorders as well as basic statistics. A 1986 study of educated, middle-class, pregnant women revealed that 25% interpreted "1 out of 1000" as 1%.

There is already a pressing need for many more professional genetic counselors to assist an overwhelming number of people to be sufficiently educated to give genuine, informed consent to testing. Careful post-screening counseling will also be needed to explain the implications of carrier status.

Wilfond and Fost calculate that in a scenario where screening is done on 3 million people annually, the required counseling time is 651,000 hours. In 1990 there were only about 450 certified genetic counselors and 500 clinical geneticists in the United States. Each one would need to devote 17 weeks of full-time work per year just to provide CF counseling.

Could public education about the importance of mass screening, even with good intentions and assuring careful counseling by experts, cause a backlash? As cystic fibrosis or any other genetic disease becomes identified as a disorder to be eliminated, how would those who choose not be be screened or who choose to bear afflicted children be regarded? Would they, for example, be threatened with loss of insurance coverage if they did not make an "acceptable" reproductive decision such as sterilization or abortion? Would they become genetic outcasts?

GENETIC DISCRIMINATION

Most humans have at least a measure of control over their daily lives. We are, as a rule, free to make choices about our education, employment, marital status, or geographical location. But we are prisoners of our genes. No one can choose his or her genetic endowment. Will the discrimination that now so often divides people based on race, dialect, gender, or physical or mental disability be extended to genetic prejudice?

Ultimately, of course, differences such as race or gender are due to one's genome. Many more subtle genome characteristics will be uncovered—such as the predisposition to heart disease, alcoholism, or mental disabilities. Perceptions may develop about people's long-term health risks and future abilities and disabilities. Will we have a new class of people who will be, as some have labeled them, the "healthy ill?"

The Council for Responsible Genetics is a Boston-based national organization of scientists, public health advocates, trade unionists, women's health activists, and others who want to see biotechnology developed safely and in the public interest. One of its fundamental goals is to work to prevent discrimination based on information generated by the increasing uses of predictive genetic tests.

The Human Genetics Committee of the council includes in its membership Ruth Hubbard, professor of Biology at Harvard University; Chairperson Paul Billings, director of the Clinic for Inherited Diseases, New England Deaconess Hospital; and Marsha Saxton, director, Project on Women and Disability. The 51-member advisory board to the council includes such well-known figures as Nobel laureates Linus Pauling and George Wald and noted ecologist Barry Commoner.

The position papers of the council concerning the HGP and genetic discrimination are good examples of articulate and informed warnings about the ethical minefields that lie ahead. They advocate a variety of steps to help circumvent these dangers with particular emphasis on preventive rather than reactive measures. Among their proposals are the encouragement of coalitions among groups concerned with civil liberties, disability rights, women's rights, procreative rights, occupational health and safety, workers' rights, and the right to health care. They urge drafting of model laws to be proposed at local, regional, state, and federal levels that would prohibit discrimination based on present or predictive medical status or hereditary traits.

Prominent among the areas of specific concern over genetic discrimination shared by most individuals and groups who have spoken and written of the subject over the last several years have been those of discimination in employment and insurance coverage. Both of these are linked by the common denominator of the ethics of privacy and confidentiality.

Employment

The Office of Technology Assessment (OTA), at the request of Congress, published a detailed report in 1983 on "The Role of Genetic Testing in the Prevention of Occupational Disease." Congress was concerned about the reports surfacing over the growing practice of genetic testing in the workplace. Incidents had been reported since the 1960s of such questionable industrial activities as programs evaluating damage to workers from exposure to chemicals or sickle-cell screening. In 1982 the OTA surveyed American industries and unions to determine the extent and nature of employer genetic testing.

Debate over whether or not such genetic testing of workers was feasible or even appropriate increased markedly during the late 1980s as new molecular genetic technology became widely available. The OTA was asked to repeat the survey. They did so in 1989 and their results and recommendations, "Genetic Monitoring and Screening in the Workplace," was published in November 1990.

The 1982 questionnaire had been sent to the 500 largest U.S. industries (Fortune 500), the 50 largest utilities, and 11 major unions. The 1989 survey covered these as well as 1000 additional companies and 22 additional unions.

The survey made a distinction between genetic monitoring and genetic screening. The former refers to a periodic examination of employees to look for changes in their genome—e.g., gross chromosomal damage or specific mutations—that might have occurred in the course of employment. The assumption is that these changes might have happened because of exposure in the workplace to hazardous substances and indicate possible increased risk of future illness. The results could indicate a need to lower exposure levels for individuals at risk.

Genetic screening involves assays that examine the genome of employees or job applicants for inherited characteristics. If such tests show susceptibility to certain occupational diseases, the company could, in the words of the OTA report, "place those workers most susceptible to a specific risk in the least hazardous environments." Screening for occupationally related traits and nonoccupationally related traits would "improve employee productivity and lower workman's compensation costs through better worker health; promote and encourage general health awareness and improve employers' health care costs . . ."

Examples of genetic factors that affect susceptibility to environmental agents are numerous. Several such conditions are, for example, the "paroxonase variant" which affects 20 to 30% of the population. It increases the risk of toxic effects due to exposure to the pesticide parathion. "Glucose-6-phosphate dehydrogenase deficiency" occurs in 16% of American males. It predisposes one to severe anemia when exposed to chemicals such as naphthalene or ozone. An "alpha-1 antitrypsin deficiency" can predispose individuals to lung disorders such as emphysema following exposure to lung irritants. This condition is the second most common type of genetic screening in U.S. industry after screening of blacks for sickle-cell trait, even though it is not at all clear that accurate predictions can be made about the risk to carriers.

Overall, the OTA found that 20 companies had used genetic monitoring or screening in 1989 as compared to 18 companies in 1982. There had supposedly been relatively little increase in the practice. In the 1989 report, 27 companies reported that they were "not sure" whether or not they would do chromosome monitoring in the next five years and 27 were "not sure" if they would do direct genetic screening. The rest said they had no such plans. The OTA concluded that their latest study "appears to indicate fewer companies anticipate using genetic monitoring or screening."

There may, in fact, be less genetic testing in industry than one might expect. However, given the employers' perspective this may be more likely due to fear of adverse publicity than an ethical decision. Certainly companies now engage in routine comprehensive testing for drugs, AIDS, high blood pressure, and so forth. They routinely give lie detector tests, handwriting analysis, and written psychological questionnaires that assess one's "honesty" or "maturity." It makes good economic sense for a company to require medical examinations for job applicants to look for the presence of diseases as well as to guard against future problems in order to reduce costs and increase productivity.

There is no reason in principle why genetic testing would not be added to the list. Corporations today often act not only as employer but as insurers and health care providers. The health of the workers ultimately affects the productivity and determines the cost of the company's health care.

One union representative who answered the 1989 OTA survey wrote "we assume that as with many other types of employer surveillance of workers genetic monitoring and screening are going on without formal notification to workers or their unions much less any request for consent."

Employers in general are regarded as being responsible for harmful affects on employees caused by their exposure to dangerous substances. Genetic screening to keep allegedly susceptible workers away from such exposure is logical. However, a major concern over genetic testing for susceptibility to harmful chemicals continues to be that it is easier and less expensive for a company to keep the workers regarded as more susceptible away from them rather than remove or modify dangerous workplace conditions. It is certainly easier to screen out all but the apparently genetically hardiest individuals than to clean up an otherwise unhealthy working environment.

Also, if employment decisions are based on genetic status, there may be illegal discrimination. Currently, there is a troublesome precedent which may interfere with defending against such discrimination. According to Dorothy Nelkin and Laurence Tancredi's 1989 book *Dangerous Diagnostics*, a 1985 code of federal regulations includes a section which requires workers to disclose "a personal history of the employee's family and occupational background including genetic and environmental factors." This rule was originally adopted in 1974 when "genetic factors" were not as readily available as they are now.

The prevention of job discrimination based on "genetic disabilities" is still problematic. Opponents of genetic testing hope to find an ally in the Americans with Disabilities Act (ADA). This legislation was finally signed into law by President Bush in 1990 after years of struggle by disabled persons intent on securing their rights of equal participation and access. The ADA extends a clear and open comprehensive prohibition of "discrimination based on disability." However, the OTA 1990 report, in referring to the ADA, said that "ADA language . . . does not specifically address genetic monitoring or screening."

However, since preemployment medical examinations can be used to determine one's ability to do the job, the OTA report does argue that "genetic screening for nonoccupationally-related conditions would seem to be prohibited." No doubt the courts will eventually be challenged to decide what role the ADA or other legislation will play in the prevention of genetic discrimination.

The international survey of medical geneticists cited earlier in connection with cystic fibrosis screening also polled attitudes toward workplace genetic screening and access to the results. Seventy-two percent were of the opinion that genetic screening in the workplace should be voluntary and 81% percent said that employers should have access to the results with the worker's consent. Twenty percent held that employers should not have any access at all. Only 6% thought that working conditions would be improved, rather than just keeping suspected susceptible individuals away from a harmful working environment.

The problems that we face in the future with regard to genetic discrimination in employment can be epitomized by some of the conclusions reached in the 262-page 1990 OTA report: "There is no consensus about how ethical issues related to genetic monitoring or screening in the workplace should be decided or whether any groups' particular interests override another's . . . it is not clear how conflicts of interest should be resolved and there is little agreement about whether workplace hazard removal should be accomplished by denying employment to genetically susceptible individuals. For now, ethical questions surrounding genetic monitoring and screening in the workplace can only be answered on a case-by-case basis."

The OTA report is detailed and generally quite objective. However, it is interesting and disturbing to note how subliminal perceptions intrude even into such a matter-of-fact document. In the first paragraph of their summary the authors refer to genetic monitoring and screening as ways to "identify *outwardly healthy* individuals (or populations) at risk for or susceptible to a variety of work-related conditions" (italics mine). In the second paragraph they refer to the great potential that these techniques have "to identify genetic abnormalities whether they be associated with inherited disease, susceptibilities and traits in *otherwise healthy* asymptomatic individuals" (italics mine). Again, are people who someday may become ill already regarded even unconsciously as the "healthy ill?"

Insurance

The basic concept behind the business of health insurance is to invite large numbers of people to pay a relatively modest fee into a pool from which those among the contributors unlucky enough to become ill can draw to cover their medical expenses. In order to improve their odds insurers routinely exclude or charge very high rates to people with preexisting conditions such as Huntington's disease, Down's syndrome, or spina bifida.

Before the age of genetic medicine both the insurer and the insured knew no more about their medical profile than they could gather from a typical medical examination. As genetic information and prediction becomes attainable and accurate, will it prove too strong a temptation for insurance companies to use genetic screening to set higher rates or deny coverage altogether for the "genetically unlucky?"

Even if legislation were passed that declared that one's genome is private and that no one can examine it without consent, that problem could be circumvented. Discounts could be made available to those whose gene profiles were "low risk" if they would allow the insurance company to have access to this information. Insurers already offer lower rates for women because they live longer than men due in good part to their genes. They also charge less for nonsmoker policies. The logic behind this asks "why should people who take care of their health subsidize others who do not?" But we do not choose our genes.

Of course, the possibility exists that a person who had a private genetic analysis that determined that he or she was at risk for a disease could apply for large amounts of insurance with the understanding that it would eventually pay for itself. After all, people without insurance are, in effect, denied quality health care. And what recourse would there be if one were deemed "genetically uninsurable?"

Is group insurance a way out of these problems? Most health insurance and about half of life insurance is supplied by employers. The premiums are adjusted based on the previous year's payouts so that the employer, not the insurer, bears the cost. As medical costs climb and predictive genetic medicine grows, employers will be pressed to screen their employees to pinpoint who may be too costly to be allowed free coverage.

It would seem that the logical outcome of highly advanced predictive genetics would inexorably move insurance from the lottery that it now essentially is to an actuarial nightmare. Preferential treatment for known low-risk individuals would mean fewer participants, higher average rates—and the death of insurance as we know it.

The usual scenario describing this regression of insurance usually ends up at national health insurance, the ultimate pooled risk. Would the government, now paying for the medical bills of the nation look kindly on, for example, the birth of a child with a genetic disease requiring expensive treatment—a child who might have been prevented?

What is the reaction of the insurance industry to these predictions? According to a cover story in *Business Week*, the American Council of Life Insurance and Health Insurance in America acknowledges that requiring genetic tests "would produce a fire storm of criticism" if it "prevented significant numbers of applicants from getting insurance at affordable rates." Robert Waldron, director of the council's New York office, put it this way: "The issue is too hot to handle."

In the 1989 international survey of medical geneticists cited earlier, 40% of the respondents thought that insurance companies should have no access at all to genetic test information even with the worker's consent.

Only 4% thought that workers would benefit in any way from an insurer knowing these results and, in fact, 30% were of the opinion that the information would be misused. Many pointed out that "access with consent" puts a person in a no-win fix—if the person denies access, he or she would probably be denied insurance.

Can abuses be prevented? According to James Watson we must legislate to make genetic discrimination illegal. "There are some things about which we must simply say you can't do it" he told geneticists at a 1990 conference in Lester, England. That argument has not worked with AIDS. Insurance companies have reacted to the spread of the virus first by demanding HIV blood tests from all single men, later denying mortgages and life insurance to those who tested positive. A positive HIV test means that the individual has been exposed to a virus that years later may cause disease. That differs little in effect from inheriting a gene that too will cause a disease later.

GENE THERAPY

It is now possible to insert genes into cells of plants, animals, and humans (see Chapter 6). Once inside the recipient cell, the genes may sometimes actually enter the genome by being spliced into a chromosome. As the cell divides, the new gene is passed from generation to generation along with the rest of the genome. The genes may begin doing the business of genes, that is, directing the production of specific proteins which play a role in the life and traits of the cell.

After years of preparation, the theory that human genes could be introduced into the cells of humans in order to correct specific genetic defects, a process called gene therapy, was finally tested in human subjects in 1990 (see Chapter 8). The early prediction that gene therapy would someday be possible had been met with skepticism and even derision. In 1968 a paper by W. French Anderson, a physician at NIH, suggesting the promise of gene therapy was rejected by the *New England Journal of Medicine* because it was "too speculative." In November 1980, Anderson and John C. Fletcher, an ethicist at NIH, published a review in the same journal on the ethical questions that this procedure would raise. Their advice has turned out to be a blueprint for the tantalizing possibilities for such genetic engineering that soon began to emerge from molecular biology laboratories. Anderson and Michael Blaese would perform the world's first human gene therapy ten years later.

Applying the familiar fundamental principle of determining in advance whether the probable benefits outweighed the probable risks, they proposed three questions that would have to be addressed using animal experimentation: (1) Can the new gene be inserted into the correct target cells so that it will remain there and be passed on to the cell descendants? (2) Will the gene product be made at an appropriate level? (3) Will the new gene harm the cell or organism?

One potential problem that could occur would be the insertion of a gene that might move into cells other than the ones intended. Or perhaps the gene could produce too much gene product and cause more harm than good. For example, a gene which stimulated insulin production too vigorously might lower blood sugar to dangerous levels. Also, since we still have many unanswered questions about how genes are "turned on" or "turned off" in cells, introduction of a new gene could unintentionally alter the genomic organization of other important genes. For example, a gene might conceivably enter a chromosome in a vital region where it might activate an oncogene, initiating the growth of a tumor.

Anderson and Fletcher pointed out that the definition of "acceptable risk" is complex. It depends in part on the severity of the patient's illness. It would have to "be so great that a potentially considerable risk from the new therapy might be justified."

Their advice and that of others has been taken seriously. Ten years later Anderson related, almost plaintively, in *Hastings Center Report* that the approval granted to the protocol that he and his colleagues had developed for their gene therapy proposal had "received the most thorough review of a clinical protocol in history." It was approved only after being reviewed 15 times by seven different regulatory bodies.

In fact, one colleague, R. Michael Blaese, remarked that "in the future if it takes all of the redundant review and such a long time as it did for us the process will have broken down. The fundamental questions have been answered." The ramifications of gene therapy, at least in this case, have received the serious attention that they deserve.

The question of balancing known specific benefits and uncertain harm was examined in detail by deliberative bodies throughout the 1980s such as the United Council of Churches, the Parliamentary Assembly of the Councils of Europe, the Medical Research Councils of Canada, the Office of Technology Assessment, and numerous others. A consensus emerged in which well-defined gene therapy based first on animal experimentation, after intensive review, should be permitted in individuals who have no other recourse.

The sex cells of the body, the sperm and the eggs, also called "gametes," are genetically distinct from all the others, the so-called "somatic cells." The sex cells each have 23 chromosomes, half the number found in the somatic cells. At fertilization the sperm and egg fuse to form a zygote which now contains the full complement of 46 chromosomes. Gene therapy in which a new gene is added to nonreproductive cells, such as blood or bone marrow cells, is referred to as somatic cell therapy. If a gene were to be added to a gamete or a fertilized egg, this would be a case of "germ-line" gene therapy.

The alluring possibility that somatic cell gene therapy may treat at least simple gene disorders like cystic fibrosis and someday perhaps multiple gene diseases such as diabetes or Alzheimer's appears to have led to its approval. The potential has outweighed the dangers of this still experimental procedure. In an interview in *Time*, Dr. Theodore Friedman, a molecular geneticist at the University of California at San Diego, reflected that "twenty years ago you couldn't utter the phrase gene therapy without being told that you were talking nonsense . . . now it's taken for granted it's coming."

GERM-LINE GENE THERAPY

The guarded optimism displayed by most commentators over somatic cell gene therapy is in strong contrast to the widespread skepticism and sometimes downright condemnation of germ-line gene therapy. Inserting genes into gametes, fertilized eggs (zygotes), or even early embryos presents a whole new set of ethical issues.

Insertion of genetic material into somatic cells is really not radically different in principle from organ transplantation or blood transfusion. But the same genes placed in a gamete, zygote, or embryo would be incorporated in all the cells of the organism which developed from them. Any trait for which a gene or genes had been isolated could then be added to a germ cell. For example, if genes for increased intelligence or disease resistance were inserted successfully into an egg, it could be fertilized in the laboratory and placed into the uterus to develop. This *in vitro* fertilization, often referred to as making "test-tube babies," is now common practice. It affords a tempting opportunity to add "desirable" genes even before fertilization.

This very scenario which makes the procedure so tempting from a strictly scientific point of view, despite the current technical obstacles, has evoked serious reservations from many sides. Could we allow the introduction of genes so early in the life of an individual that the genes would become part of every cell as that person developed through the embryo and then the fetal stage? What would be the fate of such a person if the experiment, rather than improving their life, harmed it in any way? He or she would at least be faced with the risk of passing the problem onto his or her children—if reproduction was still possible.

The European Medical Research Council representing 11 countries flatly declared in 1988 that "germ-line therapy should not be contemplated." A 1986 survey by the OTA found that only 30% of the public polled approved of the concept of attempting such a procedure. In July 1989 a symposium met in Bern, Switzerland. Scientists and philosophers, legal experts, ethicists, and theologians met to discuss the ramifications of the HGP. The mood of the meeting was, according to the chairperson Gustav Nossal, one of extraordinary caution on germ-line gene therapy. However, one year earlier at a workshop held in Valencia, Spain, French scientist Jean Dausset argued vigorously against genetic manipulation of human embryos or reproductive cells, urging geneticists not to become "sorcerers": but a motion to address the question of germ-line gene therapy in the final recommendations was not accepted.

According to Santiago Grisolia, "most scientists at the Valencia workshop considered the regulation of any experimental procedure by ethical recommendations impractical. Instead, they held a more realistic perspective that controls on genetic engineering could be imposed only by scientists themselves." To many, that is a chilling prospect.

The Council of International Organization of Medical Sciences (CIOMS) held a congress in July 1990 in Japan. The meeting was cosponsored by the World Health Organization and the United Nations Educational Scientific and Cultural Organization (UNESCO). The declaration that the council adopted represented a more positive while still cautious attitude. While openly admitting to the technical difficulties, the declaration stated that: "Continued discussion of both its (germ-line gene therapy) technical and its ethical aspects is therefore essential. Before germ-line therapy is undertaken the safety must be very well established, for changes in germ cells will affect the descendants of the patient."

ETHICS COMMITTEES

Writing on the use of genetic data, James Watson and Robert M. Cook-Deegan point out that "public policy choices have not yet been made, and there should be vigorous debate about confidentiality of genetic information, the legitimacy of various uses . . . scientists and clinicians should participate in this debate . . . coupling the scientific program to a parallel effort that assesses the broader implications of research is an unusual move for science funding agencies, but one fully justified by the history of genetics and in the face of the obvious importance of properly using human genetic information."

That is a somewhat indirect version of what Watson had said earlier that same year in a February interview in *Smithsonian*. "We have to be aware," he confessed bluntly, "of the really terrible past of eugenics . . . we have to reassure people that their own DNA is private and that no one else can get at it. We're going to have to pass laws to reassure them. [But] we don't want people rushing and passing laws without a lot of serious discussion first."

There are those who are not easily reassured. Prominent among the better known dissidents is Jeremy Rifkin, long-time activist against biotechnology. Rifkin, next to Ralph Nader, is probably the nation's best known activist against environmental neglect. He is certainly the most conspicuous enemy of genetic engineering. His Washington-based Foundation on Economic Trends has waged a war of press releases and lawsuits against, among other things: surrogate motherhood, release of genetically engineered bacteria, use of synthetic growth hormone in cattle, and gene therapy.

His flamboyant efforts have evoked reactions ranging from scathing contempt to admiration. Many scientists reluctantly allow that he asks important questions about the implications of the use of molecular genetics, but are turned off by his often shrill and vociferous opposition.

According to *Time*, Norton Zinder, a leader in the HGP, called him a "fool" and a "demagogue." Harvard's Stephen Jay Gould, a member of the advisory board of the Council for Responsible Genetics, wrote that Rifkin's popular 1983 biotech-bashing book *Algeny* was a "cleverly constructed tract of anti-intellectual propaganda masquerading as scholarship . . ."

Despite these assessments, Rifkin, sometimes referred to as the "Abominable No Man," can present positive and valid challenges. In a press release dated April 20, 1988, a national coalition of over 70 individuals and organizations, with Rifkin as spokesperson, advocated establishing a permanent congressional board and citizen's committee "to address the issues of genetic discrimination, privacy and eugenics raised by the Human Genome Project." The supporters included Ralph Nader; Molly Yard, president of the National Organization for Women; and Ed Roberts, president, World Institute on Disability.

Warning against a "new form of eugenics" Rifkin called for the establishment of a "Human Genome Policy Board" which would meet to study and report to Congress on a continuing basis "on the public policy issues . . . such as conception, education, medical and insurance coverage, and the workplace." The board would appoint a "Human Genome Advisory Committee" which would include, among others, consumer advocates, disability rights experts, and "traditional victims of past discrimination including minorities and women . . ."

The proposal was not successful, nor was a later proposal to have the NIH Recombinant DNA Advisory Committee (RAC) establish a "Human Eugenics Advisory Committee" to monitor the "ethical, philosophical, social, economic and eugenics implications of human gene therapy." However, Rifkin and his supporters did succeed in obtaining a court order on May 16, 1989 from the U.S. District Court for the District of Columbia which directed the NIH "to hold all future deliberations and votes on human gene experiments in open public session to allow for full public participation and review."

The mechanism for the "vigorous debate" called for by Watson and Cook-Deegan has taken the form of the Joint Working Group on the Ethical, Legal, and Social Issues Relative to Mapping and Sequencing the Human Genome, known, mercifully, as ELSI. Formed by the combined efforts of the National Center for Human Genome Research at NIH and the DOE Human Genome Program, ELSI is currently a six-member committee which first met in September 1989.

Our brief introduction to ethics at the beginning of this chapter suggests that their assigned task is indeed a daunting one. Critics have already taken aim at their purpose and prospects. According to columnist John Leo in *U.S. News and World Report*, "it appears as though ethicists will be cut in on some of the action and funding, as that project proceeds. But the relation of ethics to researchers is about the same as that of Army chaplain to general on the eve of an invasion. The ethicist needs to talk to the public, not the researchers."

Even more biting are the comments of Robert Wright, writer for *The New Republic*, in what amounts to a savaging of the HGP. After admitting that the funding set aside for studying these issues (an extraordinary 3% of the total budget) will allow "abundant analysis of the various policy dilemmas," he added that it will also "assure the public that everything is under control . . . (and) it can help turn down the volume of potentially voluble critics . . . it's also enough to give all the main would-be alarmists—the most likely candidates for the money, after all—a substantial interest in keeping the source of the money (the genome program) alive."

A look at the distinguished membership of ELSI should help to blunt such caustic criticism. The chairperson is Nancy Wexler, whom we have mentioned several times in connection with her pioneering work and personal experience with Huntington's disease. She is a clinical psychologist at the College of Physicians and Surgeons at Columbia University and is president of the Hereditary Disease Foundation. Members include Victor McCusick, founding president of HUGO and later chair of its ethics committee who has been a leader in the study of human genetics for over 40 years.

Jonathan R. Beckwith is a bacterial geneticist in the Department of Microbiology and Molecular Genetics at Harvard Medical School who has had a longtime concern over the ramifications of genetic screening. Dr. Robert Murray, a clinician and researcher at the Howard University College of Medicine, has been closely involved in genetic testing and screening programs, and has particular expertise on sickle-cell anemia and genetic counseling.

Attorney Patricia King has worked in civil rights law and reproductive law and has long been interested in the impact of genetic studies on minority groups. She has served on two former federal bioethics commissions as well as the NIH Recombinant DNA Advisory Committee. Attorney King was a supporter of the coalition represented by Jeremy Rifkin to establish a permanent congressional board and citizen's committee.

There is no apparent reason why the members of ELSI would have a vested interest in anything but the struggle to accomplish the aims of the ethics component of the HGP as expressed in the DOE/NIH five-year plan. Those aims are as follows:

1. Address and anticipate the implications for individuals and society of mapping and sequencing the human genome.

2. Examine the ethical, legal, and social sequelae of mapping and sequencing the human genome.

3. Stimulate public discussion of the issues.

4. Develop policy options to assure that the information is used for the benefit of the individual and society.

Faced with that task, the members of ELSI have no naiveté about the difficulty of first developing recommendations and then translating them into acceptable policies. The sixth committee member, Thomas H. Murray, director of the Center for Biomedical Ethics at Case Western Reserve University in Cleveland, warns that "it would be a terrible mistake—a pleasant delusion—to think that because we can agree on some particular policy issue we also agree on the precise moral justification for that policy . . . scratch a moral consensus and you may find a chaos of principles . . . ethics committees will have difficulty in creating policies."

ELSI's role is essentially that of initiation and coordination. Drawing on their accumulated working experience in medicine, molecular biology, genetics, psychology, and ethics they have first identified topics of particular relevance and from there are reaching out to the national and international community representing these areas of expertise and others so as to access the fullest possible participation.

The issues highlighted by ELSI will be addressed through the National Center for Human Genome Research at NIH, headed by philosopher Eric Juengst. Dr. Juengst has written to us that "The issues that will dominate the NIH first rounds of research and discussion all concern the control of predictive information about people's health. . . . Driving all of them are two values that run through almost all important questions of American social policy: privacy and the personal autonomy it provided, and social equality and the opportunity it affords. We have the moral and cultural tools to resolve these issues . . ."

According to Nancy Wexler, there are several "burning issues" which need immediate attention. These include protecting the confidentiality of genetic information, guarding against discrimination in employment and education, seeing that life and health insurance are made available to those exposed by genetic testing, and public education. She points out: "How to let people take advantage of the benefits of the genetic information, any kind of preventive or interventive medicine it may suggest, without causing them harm—I think that's really our mandate and mission."

       *   *   *

As of 1992, NIH will be investing approximately a minimum of $3–4 million annually in research grants, training grants, contracts, workshops, symposia, commissioned papers and public education. Will this unprecedented funding overcome the difficulties inherent in melding genetics, medicine, philosophy, ethics, sociology, and law into policy? The measure of success will be the emergence of a society that will apply the brilliant advances of modern science to the common good of humanity. It may well be that the most difficult task will be to agree on a definition of what that good is.

EPILOGUE

No organism except *Homo sapiens* knows anything of its history. The faint stirrings of instinct, operative in us as well, are the only vestiges within all other creatures that evoke the past. The study of history, though sometimes tedious, is likewise richly instructive. One cannot fully understand or appreciate the nature and significance of the scientific inquiry taking place within the Human Genome Project without seeing it as yet another step in a natural progression.

Increasingly detailed analyses of genomes, human and otherwise, did not arise *de novo* simply out of a desire to gain further ascendancy over our bodily functions. Such studies must be viewed in the context of that long history which we have reviewed briefly. They flow in a sometimes meandering but unbroken stream of questions posed by those dedicated to seeking their answers.

It is important to realize that the unraveling of the secrets twisted into the double helix of DNA has only just begun. The current format of that effort, which we have described in these pages as the Human Genome Project, will, in all likelihood, be altered over the remaining years of its projected 15-year existence. Discoveries will be made, technologies will improve, and attention will be diverted from one gene to another as the pieces of the mosaic fit together.

But the science will continue for now, under the rubric of the HGP and later under whatever follows. Its practitioners, the scientists, will with each advance reward the efforts of those many men and women who shaped the foundations of genetics—Gregor Mendel, Charles Darwin,

Thomas Hunt Morgan, Oswald Avery—and countless others who grappled with what were often seemingly intractable questions.

As a practicing scientist, the author can attest to the fact that, while science holds no copyright on honesty, the instances of unethical and deceptive practices in the world's scientific community are notable only as exceptions to the rule. Most scientific research is marked by an extraordinary integrity. The personalities of researchers are as diverse as any other variegated population. But despite the fact that for a few the lure of fame and moderate fortune motivates them to sometimes bitter skirmishes with their peers, the ordinary relationships among scientists are marked by acts of generosity, support, and sharing that is perhaps found in no other profession.

A pervasive sense of wonder develops as one considers the many vectors traveled over the course of the 3–4 billion years of evolution which have converged to shape human beings. It is only a scant few decades since some of those humans began to discover the molecular basis of living systems and the first rudiments of the preeminent role of DNA. Evolution, reduced to its essentials, is a series of changes in DNA, much of which disappear with the death of the cells that house it. But some altered DNA survives, replicates, and is passed on to another generation. The genes within the DNA carry the code that now, after billions of years of random but often (or so it seems to us as its heirs) fortuitous changes, translates into men and women with the intellectual powers to begin to understand how this incredible journey has occurred.

These last few pages are being written during the bicentennial of the death of Mozart. The searing beauty of his music shows the heights to which humans can soar. But on this very day the world is at war in the Middle East. The massive lobes of the cerebral cortex of our brain elevate our intelligence far beyond that of any other animal. But deep beneath the cerebrum lies our evolutionary past. We can lead loving, creative lives— and we can also kill each other in response to innate drives of aggression, territoriality, and fear which we scarcely understand. The contradictions inherent in this example give rise to the misgivings that we have discussed about the way in which the knowledge and power gained by genome analysis may be used.

Galileo asked in 1615, "Who indeed will set bounds to human ingenuity?" In the last decade of the twentieth century, ethicist John C. Fletcher would echo the same sentiment toward the tantalizing study of the human genome. "The desire to know," said Fletcher, "will transcend the fear of knowing." True to the past and true to our human nature, we will continue to learn about how this awesome universe functions, from measuring the enormous distances between galaxies to measuring the invisible molecular spaces between genes. Knowledge and wisdom are distinct. The former will grow inexorably as we continue to gain control over DNA. Will the latter keep pace?

FURTHER READING

General

Stephen S. Hall, "James Watson and the search for biology's 'Holy Grail,'" *Smithsonian* (February 1990), pp. 41–49

Victor A. McCusick, "Mapping and sequencing the human genome," *New England Journal of Medicine* (6 April, 1989), pp. 910–915

Leon Jaroff, "The gene hunt," *Time* (20 March 1989), pp. 62–67

Roger Lewin, "In the beginning was the genome," *New Scientist* (21 July, 1990), pp. 34–38

James D. Watson, "The Human Genome Project: Past, present and future," *Science* (6 April 1990), pp. 44–49

DNA History

Horace Freeland Judson, *The Eighth Day of Creation*. New York: Simon and Schuster, 1979

Anne Sayre, *Rosalind Franklin and DNA*. New York: W.W. Norton and Company, 1975

Nancy A. Tiley, *Discovering DNA: Meditations on Genetics and a History of the Science*. New York: Van Nostrand Reinhold Company, 1983

James D. Watson, *The Double Helix*. New York: Atheneum Publishers, 1968

Genetics and DNA

David T. Suzuki and Tony Griffiths, *Introduction to Genetic Analysis*, 4th ed. New York: W.H. Freeman, 1989

Newsletters and Journals

Betty K. Mansfield, ed., *Human Genome News* (Oak Ridge National Laboratory, P.O. Box 2008, Oak Ridge, Tennessee 37831-6050)

Victor A. McCusick and Frank H. Ruddle, eds., *Genomics: International Journal of Gene Mapping and Nucleotide Sequencing Emphasizing Analyses of the Human and Other Complex Genomes.* Duluth, Minnesota: Academic Press

Genome Mapping and Sequencing

Mapping and Sequencing the Human Genome. Washington, D.C.: National Academy Press, 1988

Mapping Our Genes: Genome Projects: How Big, How Fast? Baltimore: The Johns Hopkins University Press, 1988

Understanding Our Genetic Inheritance: The U.S. Human Genome Project: The First Five Years FY 1991–1995. Springfield, Virginia: National Technical Information Service, 1990

Ray White and Jean-Marc Lalouel, "Chromosome mapping with DNA markers," *Scientific American* (February 1988) **258**:40–48

Avril D. Woodhead and Benjamin J. Barnhart, eds., *Biotechnology and the Human Genome: Innovations and Impact.* New York: Plenum Press, 1988

Ethics and Law

George J. Annas, "Mapping the human genome and the meaning of monster mythology," *Emory Law Journal* (Summer 1990) **39**:629–642

Sherman Elias and George J. Annas, *Reproductive Genetics and the Law.* Chicago, Illinois: Year Book Medical Publishers, 1987

Szolt Harsanyi and Richard Hutton, *Genetic Prophecy: Beyond the Double Helix.* New York: Rawson, Wade Publishers, 1981

Marc Lappé, *Broken Code: The Exploitation of DNA.* San Francisco: Sierra Club Books, 1984

Aubrey Milunskey and George J. Annas, eds., *Genetics and the Law III.* New York: Plenum Press, 1985

Dorothy Nelkin and Laurence Tancredi, *Dangerous Diagnostics.* New York: Basic Books, 1989

Charles Piller and Keith R. Yamamoto, *Gene Wars: Military Control Over the New Genetic Technologies.* New York: Beech Tree Books–William Morrow, 1988

Jeremy Rifkin, *Algeny.* New York: The Viking Press, 1983

David Suzuki, *Genetics: The Clash between the New Genetics and Human Values.* Cambridge, Massachusetts: Harvard University Press, 1989

Burke K. Zimmerman, *Biofuture: Confronting the Genetic Era.* New York: Plenum Press, 1984

Eugenics

Daniel J. Kevles, *In the Name of Eugenics: Genetics and the Uses of Human Heredity.* Berkeley, California: University of California Press, 1985

J. David Smith, *Minds Made Feeble: The Myth and Legacy of the Kallikaks.* Rockville, Maryland: Aspen, 1985

Genes and Disease

Jared Diamond, "The cruel logic of our genes," *Discover* (November 1989), pp. 72–78

Denise Grady, "The ticking of a time bomb in the genes," *Discover* (June 1987), pp. 26–39

Genetic Screening

David Beers, "The gene screen," *Vogue* (June 1990), pp. 236–237, 278–279

"The telltale gene," *Consumer Reports* (July 1990), pp. 483–488

Christopher Joyce, "Your genome in their hands," *New Scientist* (11 August 1990), pp. 52–55

Mark A. Rothstein, *Medical Screening and the Employee Health Cost Crisis.* Washington, D.C.: BNA Books, 1984

U.S. Congress, Office of Technology Assessment, *Genetic Monitoring and Screening in the Workplace*, OTA-BA-455. Washington, D.C.: U.S. Government Printing Office, 1990

Gene Therapy

Joan O. C. Hamilton and Naomi Freundlich, "The genetic age," *Business Week* (28 May, 1990), pp. 68–83

Geoffrey Montgomery, "The ultimate medicine," *Discover* (March 1990), pp. 60–68

Inder M. Verma, "Gene therapy," *Scientific American* (November 1990), pp. 68–84

GLOSSARY

Allele: A particular form of a gene at a gene locus on a chromosome.

Amino Acid: Any one of 20 molecules that can combine in many different sequences to make a wide variety of proteins.

Autosome: A chromosome not used for sex determination. The human genome is made up of 22 pairs of autosomes and 1 pair of sex chromosomes.

Bacteriophage: A virus that infects bacteria.

Biotechnology: Any technology that uses living organisms or parts of organisms to make or modify products to improve plants or animals or to develop microorganisms for specific uses.

Carrier: A person who carries a particular gene within his or her genome where it remains essentially inactive. The gene may be passed on to an offspring in which, because of the presence of another gene contributed by the other parent, it may express itself as a trait.

Centimorgan: A unit to express crossing-over frequency. One centimorgan is equal to a 1% crossover frequency between two locations on a chromosome.

Chromosome: The structure in the cell that carries the genes. These structures appear through the microscope as small rods. They are made up of DNA and proteins. In bacteria they are circular strands.

Cloning: The production of multiple copies of a cell or its DNA.

Complementary DNA (cDNA): DNA that is made using complementary RNA. In its single-stranded form cDNA is often used as a probe.

Contigs: Groups of DNA clones that are overlapping (contiguous) regions of a genome.

Crossing-Over: The exchange of chromosome segments by breakage and reunion during meiosis.

Diploid: A full set of chromosomes, half from each parent. The human diploid number is 46.

DNA: Deoxyribonucleic acid; the genetic material of living organisms. It exists in cells as a double helix.

Dominant: An allele whose effect is often the same in the heterozygous and homozygous condition.

Double Helix: The configuration of the DNA molecule. Two strands of nucleotides wrap around each other to form the double helix, which is that shape of uniform diameter that would result from wrapping two wires around a cylinder.

Drosophila: The scientific name for a particular type of fruit fly widely used in genetics research.

Electrophoresis: A method of separating molecules. They travel along an electric current in a medium (often a gel) at different rates depending on their charge and size.

Embryo: The early developmental stage of an organism developing from a fertilized egg. In the case of humans, this refers to the first two months of life in the uterus.

Enzyme: A protein that speeds up a chemical reaction in a cell.

Eugenics: Attempts to improve human inheritance by some form of genetic control such as selective breeding

Exon: That part of the DNA that actually has a code for protein synthesis.

Fetus: The developing human organism during the last seven months of prenatal life.

Gamete: A sexual reproductive cell. In humans it is either a sperm or egg cell. Both are haploid.

Gene: A specific sequence of nucleotides in a DNA molecule that has the code for the synthesis of a specific polypeptide.

Gene Therapy: The insertion of normal genes into human cells in an attempt to overcome the effects of defective genes.

Genetic Linkage Map: A map of the relative positions of genes or other identifiable genetic markers on a chromosome. It is made by determining how often the genes or markers are inherited together.

Genetic Monitoring: An examination of genomes at intervals in order to look for changes in those genomes over a period of time.

Genetic Screening: Examining genomes in order to look for inherited characteristics.

Genetics: The study of the inheritance of specific traits.

Genome: The complete complement of an organism's genes; an organism's genetic material.

Germ-Line Gene Therapy: Inserting normal genes into gametes or fertilized eggs in an attempt either to correct a genetic defect or to improve the genome.

Haploid: A half set of chromosomes. The haploid number in human cells is 23.

Heterozygous: Having two different alleles at the same locus on a pair of homologous chromosomes.

Homologous: Refers to chromosome pairs that carry genes for the same characteristics at the same site on each chromosome. The genes may be the same or different.

Homozygous: Having two identical alleles at the same locus on a pair of homologous chromosomes.

Introns: The DNA sequences that are translated into messenger RNA but are then cut out because they do not have a code for protein synthesis.

Karyotype: A photographic display of the number, shapes, and sizes of an organism's chromosomes.

Library: A collection of DNA clones whose relationships can be established by physical mapping.

Linkage: DNA segments, such as genes or RFLP markers, that are on the same chromosome and hence will be inherited together unless separated by crossing-over.

Locus: A specific site on a chromosome.

Marker: An identifiable part of a chromosome whose inheritance can be followed. Examples are restriction enzyme cutting sites, RFLP markers, or genes.

Meiosis: The form of cell division in which the diploid number is reduced to the haploid number, resulting in 4 haploid gametes.

Messenger RNA (mRNA): A type of RNA made by transcribing a sequence of nucleotides (a gene) in DNA. It moves to the ribosome where it passes on the code for making a polypeptide.

Mitosis: The form of cell division in which the chromosome number is duplicated, resulting in two identical cells.

Mutation: A change in a DNA nucleotide sequence. If such a change occurs in a sexually reproductive cell, the change may be passed on.

Nitrogenous Base: A nitrogen-containing molecule. Four types of these bases are in DNA: adenine (A), thymine (T), guanine (G), and cytosine (C). A fifth, uracil (U), is in RNA instead of thymine.

Nucleotide: The building blocks of DNA and RNA, made up of a nitrogenous base, a five-carbon sugar, and a phosphate group.

Nucleus: The structure in the center of the cell which houses the chromosomes.

Oligonucleotide: A short chain of nucleotides of known nitrogenous base sequence which can be synthesized in the laboratory.

Oncogene: A gene associated with the development of cancer.

PCR: Polymerase chain reaction. A laboratory procedure in which minute quantities of DNA can be copied millions of times in a few hours.

Physical Map: A map of the markers on DNA, regardless of inheritance. The distance between the sites is measured in nitrogenous base pairs.

Plasmid: A small, circular DNA molecule in bacterial cells. Plasmids are used in recombinant DNA procedures to pick up and carry foreign DNA into cells.

Polygenic: A characteristic controlled by more than one pair of genes.

Polypeptide: A strand of amino acids. Several polypeptides combine to make a protein.

Primer: An oligonucleotide used to attach to a complementary stretch of DNA. This can "prime" or start further synthesis of that DNA, such as in PCR.

Probe: Molecules, often single-stranded DNA, that are used to attach to complementary nitrogenous base sequences to identify their location, e.g., after electrophoresis.

Protein: A large molecule, usually made up of several linked polypeptides.

Recessive: An allele whose effect may be masked by the presence of a dominant allele on the other homologous chromosome.

Recombinant DNA: DNA that is put together in the laboratory by combining DNA fragments from several organisms. It can be introduced into cells where it may be functional.

Replication: The synthesis of new DNA from existing DNA. The double helix opens and each side acts as a template for the synthesis of a new complementary strand.

Restriction Enzyme: An enzyme isolated from bacteria that recognizes specific DNA nucleotide sequences and cuts the DNA at that site.

Restriction Fragment Length Polymorphism: Also known as RFLP. Variation in the size of DNA fragments cut by restriction enzymes. The nucleotide sequences that are responsible for RFLPs are useful as markers in constructing genetic linkage maps.

RNA: Ribonucleic acid. It is active in protein synthesis in three forms, messenger, transfer, and ribosomal RNA.

Sequence: To determine the specific order of nitrogenous bases in DNA or RNA or that of amino acids in a protein.

Sex-Linked: An inherited trait determined by a gene on a sex chromosome.

Sticky Ends: Exposed, unpaired nitrogenous bases extending from the end of a DNA molecule. These are used in recombinant DNA to recombine DNA from different sources.

STS: A sequence tagged site. A short stretch of DNA with a known nitrogenous base sequence used as a marker in physical mapping of genomes.

YAC: Yeast artificial chromosome. A new piece of DNA is spliced into a yeast chromosome and used in mapping genomes. YACs are large, up to more than a half-million base pairs long.

INDEX

Abbe, Ernst, 39
Abortion
    ethics, 260, 270–275
    genetic screening and, 17
    numbers performed, 270
Adenosine deaminase deficiency (ADA),
        genetic therapy for, 202–204
Agarose, gel electrophoresis and, 136–
        137
Agent Orange, 211
Agriculture
    genetic research and, 33
    origins of, 22
AIDS
    polymerase chain reaction and, 145
    research approaches and, 244
    research costs for, 225, 249
    retroviruses and, 133
Alta, conference, 8–9, 210–211
Alzheimer's disease, health applications,
        194–195
Americans with Disabilities Act of 1990,
        286
Amici, Giovanni, 39
Amino acids
    DNA molecule and, 78–79
    proteins and, 90, 92, 95–100
Anderson, W. French, 289–290
Annas, George J., 231–232, 240, 261,
        277

Aristotle, 24
Asilomar Conference recommendations,
        118
Atomic bomb, 210
Australia, 251
Automation, Human Genome Project
        and, 13–14, 174–176
Avery, Oswald, 65, 67, 68, 300

Bacteria
    cloning of, 112
    genetic research and, 65–68, 87–88,
        91–92
    plasmids research and, 112–117
    procaryotic cell, 126
    virus infection of, 69–72, 82, 104
Bacteriophage, 69–72, 82, 104
Baltimore, David, 10, 133, 224
Barker, Robert, 240
Barnett, Leslie, 98
Bases, nitrogenous, 4, 79–87
Bateson, William, 21, 51, 56, 61, 67
Beadle, George, 62, 63, 64
Beall, Robert, 271
Beckwith, Jonathan R., 296
Berg, Paul, 106, 114, 118, 216
Bergson, Henri, 24
Big science criticism, discussed, 237–
        242
Billings, Paul, 282

313